Self-Assessment Color Review of
Small Animal Emergency & Critical Care Medicine

Rebecca Kirby
DVM DACVIM DACVECC
Animal Emergency Center
Milwaukee, USA

Iowa State University Press/Ames

Broad Classification of Cases

Cardiovascular
29, 39, 51, 57, 65, 68, 75, 79, 92, 102, 106, 111, 121, 131, 142, 154, 165, 169, 180, 195, 220

Respiratory
3, 7, 8, 15, 30, 36, 49, 55, 62, 73, 76, 82, 84, 95, 103, 118, 126, 145, 146, 149, 156, 171, 193, 199, 202, 206, 211, 216

Urinary
13, 46, 48, 104, 116, 122, 161, 172, 173, 180, 183, 189

Gastrointestinal
23, 24, 44, 52, 54, 74, 83, 91, 95, 99, 106, 117, 125, 132, 147, 150, 158, 178, 200

Reticuloendothelial system
26, 50, 77, 78, 87, 97, 114

Endocrine
34, 40, 42, 67, 110, 151, 194

Toxins
2, 58, 71, 134, 148, 150, 180

Reproduction
16, 35, 61, 100, 136, 155, 168, 179

Feline
26, 40, 42, 50, 62, 76, 88, 98, 110, 116, 119, 211

Ophthalmology
5, 11, 33, 53, 81, 104, 107, 143, 160

Surgical
3, 9, 22, 25, 31, 63, 72, 78, 95, 96, 99, 114, 115, 117, 120, 123, 127, 132, 136, 139, 141, 161, 174, 176, 178, 187, 196, 197, 212, 222

Trauma
4, 6, 9, 20, 25, 30, 31, 36, 45, 48, 62, 63, 66, 68, 70, 95, 96, 105, 114, 115, 120, 123, 127, 128, 156, 176, 199, 203, 204, 210

First aid and transport
6, 11, 32, 47, 108, 127, 144, 152, 163, 188, 195

Fluid and electrolytes
1, 4, 3, 28, 60, 70, 87, 88, 91, 98, 110, 113, 153, 166, 182, 183, 185, 186, 189, 194, 201, 205, 209, 210

Anesthesia/analgesia
3, 64, 80, 86, 96, 137, 140, 145

Neurology
4, 19, 21, 37, 41, 80, 89, 93, 124, 165, 166, 167, 184, 219, 220

Shock
4, 51, 60, 62, 66, 71, 74, 88, 90, 101, 128, 144, 169, 170, 190, 191

Polysystemic disease
12, 15, 17, 29, 38, 52, 86, 135, 157, 159, 164, 170, 175

Orthopedic
14, 19, 20, 56, 62, 105, 138, 207, 208, 213, 215

Hematology
7, 10, 12, 18, 27, 38, 59, 69, 73, 85, 112, 118, 133, 162, 177, 179, 192, 198, 214

Nutrition
43, 52, 109

Abbreviations used in the book are given on page 189.

First published in the United States of America in 1998 by
Iowa State University Press, 2121 South State Avenue, Ames, Iowa 50014-8300
ISBN: 0-8138-2959-3

Copyright © 1998 Manson Publishing Ltd
73 Corringham Road, London NW11 7DL, UK.
All rights reserved. No part of this publication may be reproduced, stored in a retrieval system or transmitted in any form or by any means without the writtenpermission of the copyright holder or in accordance with the provisions of the Copyright Act 1956 (as amended), or under the terms of any licence permitting limited copying issued by the Copyright Licensing Agency, 33–34 Alfred Place, London WC1E 7DP.

Any person who does any unauthorised act in relation to this publication may be liable to criminal prosecution and civil claims for damages.

A CIP catalogue record for this book is available from the British Library.

Text editing: Peter Beynon
Design and layout: Patrick Daly
Project management: John Ormiston
Color reproduction: Reed Digital, Ipswich, UK
Printed by: Grafos SA, Barcelona, Spain

Preface

It's 2AM and you have just finished a gastropexy on a standard poodle that is now experiencing ventricular premature contractions. The diabetic cat that has insulin overdose is beginning to twitch and there is a male orange-and-white cat waiting to have its urethra unblocked. Your technician relays to you that there are four different animals on their way in to see you: two hit by cars, one near drowning, and one big dog–little dog fight. Your catecholamines are at an all-time high. This is why you love your work!

The *Self-Assessment Color Review of Small Animal Emergency and Critical Care Medicine* provides a challenging and entertaining mechanism for expanding medical and surgical skills in this specialty. Over 20 veterinarians have been selected to contribute to this text. Most authors are diplomates of the American College of Veterinary Emergency and Critical Care, and the others are highly respected veterinarians practicing state-of-the-art emergency medicine from countries around the world. The cases and questions presented demonstrate important principles and provide pearls from experience intended to contribute to successful patient management.

The reader is encouraged to work alone or with a group of colleagues and test their skills. Read the case history and prepare your answer before reading the suggestions from the authors. We present what we believe is our best answer. However, there is often more than one technique for carrying out a procedure or more than one approach to diagnosing and treating a patient. We hope you are stimulated to study physiology, internal medicine, surgery, and emergency medicine texts for more complete explanations and additional therapeutic options.

Medicine, surgery, anesthesia, clinical pathology, radiology, neurology, cardiology ... you have to know it all in emergency and critical care medicine. The right decision must be made at the right time. The staff and equipment must be in readiness for multiple animals with any possible crisis. The ups and downs of this specialty will remind you of a high speed roller coaster ride.

So, sit down, buckle up ... and get ready for the ride of your life!

Rebecca Kirby
DVM DACVIM DACVECC

Acknowledgments

The compilation of emergency and critical care cases published herein is the result of many hours of hard work by the contributors and publisher's staff. I am very grateful for and acknowledge their talents, skills, and dedication. Each individual contribution has made this book accurate, coherent, and easy to read. The staff at Manson Publishing have edited the questions to a reasonable text length (an enormous amount of work) and provided both American units and European units. Thus, this book is of benefit to everyone in the veterinary profession worldwide. Thank you very much for a job done with excellence.

Rebecca Kirby
DVM DACVIM DACVECC

Contributors

Linda Barton DACVECC
The Animal Medical Center
New York, NY, USA

Peter GC Bedford
BVetMed, PhD, FRCVS
Royal Veterinary College
Hatfield, UK

Jennifer Brinson
University of Missouri
Columbia, MO, USA

Claudio Brovida DVM
ANUBI Companion Animals Hospital
Moncalieri, Torino, Italy

Jennifer Devey DVM,
DACVECC
SouthPaws Veterinary Referral Center
Springfield, VA, USA

Kenneth J Drobatz DVM,
DACVECC, DACVIM
University of Pennsylvania
Philadelphia, PA, USA

Nishi Dupa DACVECC,
DACVIM
Tufts University
North Grafton, MA, USA

Ava Firth DVM, MVS,
DACVECC
University of Melbourne
VIC, Australia

Roger Gfeller DVM,
DACVECC
Veterinary Emergency Services Inc
Fresno, CA, USA

Ludo J Hellebrekers Dipl
ECVA
University of Utrecht
Utrecht, The Netherlands

Karin Holler IVECCS, EUFM,
AAFP
Tierklinik Leonding
Leonding, Austria

Justine A Johnson DVM,
DACVECC
Tufts University
North Grafton, MA, USA

Rebecca Kirby DVM,
DACVIM, DACVECC
Animal Emergency Center
Milwaukee, WI, USA

Douglass K Macintire
DVM, MS, DACVIM,
DACVECC
Auburn University
Auburn, AL, USA

Fred Anthony Mann DVM,
MS, DACVS, DACVECC
University of Missouri–Columbia
Columbia, MO, USA

Karol A Mathews DVM,
DVSc, DACVECC
University of Guelph
Ontario, Canada

Rob Moreau DVM,
DACVECC
Beach Animal Hospital and Specialty Services
Point Pleasant Beach, NJ, USA

Erika Mueller DVM
Veterinary Referral and Emergency Center
Norwalk, CT, USA

Robert J Murtaugh DVM,
MS, DACVIM, DACVECC
Tufts University
North Grafton, MA, USA

Yonathan Peres DVM
The Hebrew University of Jerusalem
Rehovot, Israel

Deanna Purvis VMD,
DACVECC
SouthPaws Veterinary Referral Center
Springfield, VA, USA

Angel Rivera AHT, CVT
Animal Emergency Center
Milwaukee, WI, USA

Joris H Robben DVM,
DECVIM
University of Utrecht
Utrecht, The Netherlands

Elke Rudloff DVM,
DACVECC
Animal Emergency Center
Milwaukee, WI, USA

Bill Saxon DVM, DACVIM,
DACVECC
Grafton, CA, USA

David Spreng DVM, DECVS
University of Bern
Bern, Switzerland

Debbie Van Pelt DACVECC
Colorado State University
Fort Collins, CO, USA

1–3: Questions

1 A three-year-old, spayed female dog (1) is presented for depression, lethargy and polyuria/polydipsia. Blood tests find: Ca^{++} (total) – 19.32 mg/dl (4.83 mmol/l); phosphorus – 7.73 mg/dl (2.48 mmol/l); PCV* – 48%; TS – 7.0 g/dl.
i. The differential diagnosis for this dog's hypercalcemia includes all of the following except for:
a. Vitamin D toxicosis.
b. Hypercalcemia of malignancy.
c. Ethylene glycol intoxication.
d. Primary hyperparathyroidism.
e. Severe hypothermia.
ii. Appropriate fluid therapy consists of all of the following except for:
a. Fluid diuresis with normal saline.
b. Furosemide administration.
c. Hydrochlorthiazide administration.
d. Prednisolone.
iii. Is there a concern for tissue mineralization in this dog?
iv. The mechanism of the polyuria and polydypsia in this dog is:
a. Direct stimulation of the thirst center.
b. Interference with antidiuretic hormone in the collecting tubules.
c. Tubulointerstitial injury.
d. All of the above.

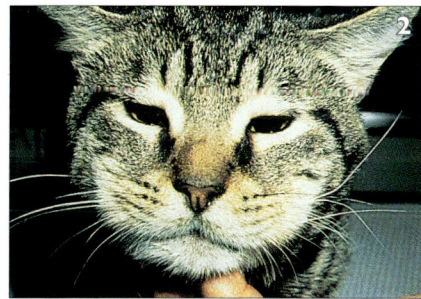

2 A three-year-old cat is presented because of lethargy, rapid respirations and brown mucous membranes (2). On physical examination the cat is hypersalivating, has facial edema, and is tachypneic and tachycardic. Upon placement of an i/v catheter, the blood is dark brown.
i. What is the most likely cause of this cat's clinical signs?
ii. What is the mechanism of action of this toxin?
iii. What cells in the body are mainly affected in the cat and in the dog?
iv. What are the specific treatments for this intoxication?

3 A three-year-old Afghan Hound presents with a torsion of the right middle lung lobe.
i. What type of analgesic regimen should be considered in this patient from the moment of entry into the hospital to the time of discharge?
ii. Briefly describe the surgical technique for treating this disease.
iii. What complications should be anticipated intraoperatively?
iv. How should this patient be managed postoperatively?

*Abbreviations used in this book are given on page 189.

1–3: Answers

1 i. c.
ii. c.
iii. When the product of the calcium and phosphorus is greater than 70, there is tissue mineralization and possible renal damage. This dog's product is 149, i.e. 19.32 × 7.73.
iv. d.

2 i. Acetaminophen intoxication. The owner should be questioned regarding the cat's potential exposure to medicine containing this drug, e.g. cold remedies or aspirin-free analgesics.
ii. Oxidative stress to the RBCs and hepatocytes. Cytochrome P-450 mediated oxidation produces a toxic metabolite that can cause: a. RBC glutathione binding, causing methemoglobinemia; b. hepatotoxicity in a dose-dependent manner.
iii. RBCs in the cat, causing methemoglobinemia and Heinz body formation. Hepatocytes are more affected in the dog.
iv. Emesis and activated charcoal if within 4–6 hours of ingestion. Oxygen and i/v fluids. N-acetylcysteine (140 mg/kg i/v followed by 70 mg/kg po 4 times daily for 7 treatments); ascorbic acid (30 mg/kg po or s/c). Methylene blue (1–2 mg/kg i/v) for emergency conversion of methemoglobin to hemoglobin. Watch for Heinz bodies. Cimetadine (10 mg/kg i/v, im, po q6–8h).

3 i. A thoracocentesis can generally be performed without analgesia; however, if the patient has recently sustained trauma to the chest, a local anesthetic block with lidocaine should be considered prior to performing the thoracocentesis. The patient should receive pre-emptive analgesia using systemic narcotics. An intercostal nerve block using bupivacaine will also help with pain management if performed pre-emptively, and can be repeated during the postoperative period. The intercostal nerves to the ribs immediately cranial and caudal to the thoracotomy site, as well as the nerves to the rib space involved in the surgery, are blocked. Postoperatively, bupivacaine can be infused into the chest tube.
ii. A lateral thoracotomy is performed on the affected side with the incision centered over the affected lung. Lung lobes may be adhered to the pleura, therefore the pleural space is entered carefully to avoid lacerating the lung. The lung lobe is removed in the twisted position to prevent release of inflammatory mediators from the hypoxic lung tissue into the systemic circulation. A total lobectomy is performed. The lobe can be resected using a stapling device (TA55) or sutures. If using sutures, the bronchus is oversewn using single interrupted sutures, and the artery and vein are transfixed or double ligated using nonabsorbable suture. A 5 mm section of vessel is left beyond each ligature. If possible, the artery, vein and bronchus are ligated separately. If there is any restrictive pleuritis involving the other lobes, the fibrin is peeled away. The chest is lavaged and a chest tube (same diameter as main bronchus) is placed. The chest is closed in a routine fashion.
iii. Manipulation of the torsed lung may cause an intense vagal response and atropine may be required. Hypotension secondary to anesthetic agents and inflammatory mediators from the lung may occur. Lungs may bleed significantly as fibrin is peeled away.
iv. Supplemental oxygen, i/v fluids, antibiotics and analgesics should be provided. A chest tube will be required postoperatively for 12–48 hours. This should be suctioned frequently (hourly) initially, then as needed. Fluid cytology should be evaluated every 24–48 hours for signs of infection. Albumin levels and coagulation parameters should also be monitored. Enteral nutrition should be started as soon possible.

4–6: Questions

4 This three-year-old cat presented 30 minutes after falling out of a ninth-storey window (4). Your primary survey reveals: HR – 160 bpm; normal lung sounds with panting; gum color is pale with a 2–3 second CRT; femoral pulses are weak; anisocoria and decreased mentation; blood noted in the nose, mouth and left ear.
i. What stage of shock (compensatory, early decompensatory, decompensatory) is this patient in? Justify the selection.
ii. Considering the choices of fluid for resuscitation:
a. Comment on the use of hypertonic saline or mannitol in this patient.
b. Comment on the use of hetastarch in this patient.
c. Comment on the use of Dextran-40 in this patient.
iii. This cat's BP increased from 100/70 to 150/100 mmHg (13.3/9.3 to 20/13.3 kPa) during the resuscitation. Is there any concern with this development?
iv. What is the ultimate goal with fluid resuscitation of a patient with head injuries?

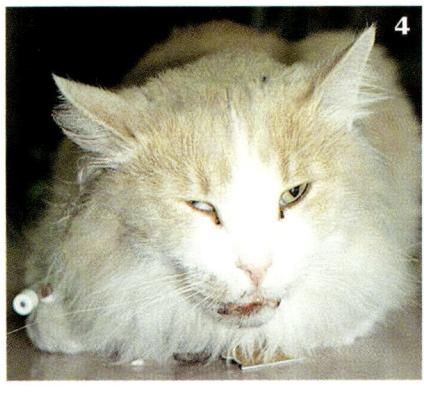

5 A seven-year-old Welsh Springer Spaniel presented with acute onset unilateral (left) ocular pain, witnessed by blepharospasm, excessive lacrimation and photophobia. Initial examination revealed marked episcleral congestion, a mild corneal edema and a dilated (light non-responsive) pupil (5).
i. What is your diagnosis?
ii. What would you expect to find on tonometry?
iii. What would gonioscopic examination of the right eye most likely reveal?
iv. How would you treat this patient?

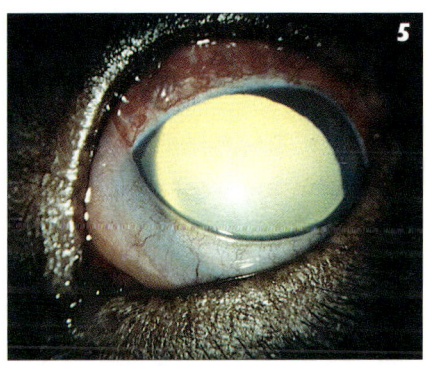

6 The owner calls you about this cat (6) which was hit by a car and is in obvious respiratory distress.
i. What are your recommendations for transport?
ii. What parameters should be monitored during transport?
iii. How do you prepare the hospital and staff prior to presentation?

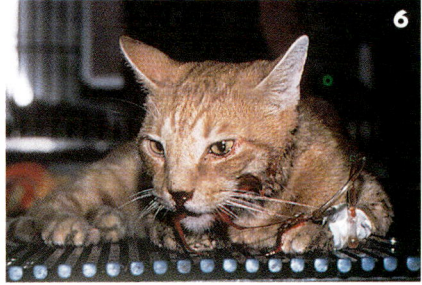

4–6: Answers

4 i. Early decompensatory stage.
ii. a. Intracranial hemorrhage is possible in this case. Hypertonic solutions such as hypertonic saline and mannitol are controversial for treatment because they can leak into the brain tissue, exacerbating hemorrhage and ICP.
b. Hetastarch in modest amounts would decrease the volume of fluid required for maintaining cerebral perfusion pressure. However, should hetastarch leak into the brain parenchyma from a damaged vessel, edema and increased ICP can result.
c. Dextran-40 coats platelets. For this reason it is not the fluid of choice in the bleeding patient because it may decrease hemostasis.
iii. Cerebral hypertension can cause increased bleeding and edema into the cranium, worsening the situation. It can also lower cerebral perfusion pressure.
iv. To promote cerebral perfusion without increasing ICP.

5 i. Primary angle-closure glaucoma.
ii. A high intraocular pressure.
iii. Goniodysgenesis in which the entrance to the ciliary cleft would be narrowed, i.e. a narrow angle.
iv. The intraocular pressure must be reduced as soon as possible. Emergency therapy is based on the use of an hyperosmotic agent, e.g. i/v mannitol or oral glycerol. Long-term intraocular pressure control necessitates the use of bypass (shunt) surgery or laser photocoagulation of the ciliary body.

6 i. Transport must be immediate. Avoid stressing the cat and use minimal restraint. If there is evidence of airway obstruction try to clear the back of the throat. Apply direct pressure over any bleeding area. If the owner has access to oxygen, direct the hose toward the mouth or nose, or direct it into the box or carrier after the door has been covered.
ii. Respiratory rate and effort, gum color, level of consciousness and occurrence of bleeding.
iii. The receptionist notifies the veterinarian and nursing staff of the impending arrival. The nursing staff lays out the following:
• *Airway* – small endotracheal tubes with air-filled syringes; gauze to tie in the tube; laryngoscope with small blade; suction unit with small tip.
• *Breathing* – AMBU bag; oxygen source; nasal catheter setup; materials for emergency chest tap and chest tube placement; drugs for sedation and pain relief.
• *Circulation* – i/v or i/o catheters; tape; clippers; heparinized flush; crystalloids.

7 & 8: Questions

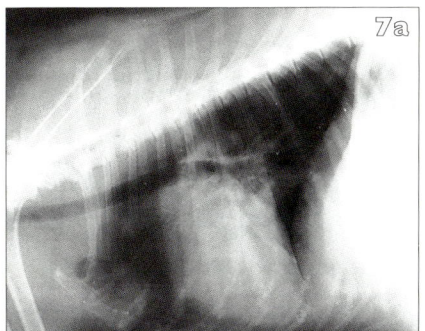

7 An eight-year-old, spayed female Cocker Spaniel has been hospitalized for one week undergoing therapy for immune-mediated hemolytic anemia. Her PCV is rising slowly and her serum is less icteric, but you notice a dramatic increase in respiratory effort this morning. Thoracic radiographs are taken (7a, 7b).
i. Describe the radiographic findings.
ii. An arterial blood gas assessment reveals a PaO_2 of 45 mmHg (normal 85–105 mmHg; 6.0 kPa, normal 11.3–14 kPa) and a $PaCO_2$ of 39 mmHg (normal 30–44 mmHg; 5.2 kPa, normal 4.0–5.9 kPa). What is the probable diagnosis?
iii. How could you confirm the diagnosis?
iv. How would you treat this condition?

8 Acute respiratory distress in the dog and cat presents as a life-threatening emergency. Performing aggressive diagnostic tests can lead to rapid decompensation and death. It is critical to employ careful observation of the animal's breathing pattern and effort to localize where the pathology lies and to determine the degree of severity.
i. Cyanosis is a late sign of respiratory compromise. List in order the changes that can be observed as they occur in the dog and cat with progressive respiratory compromise.
ii. Describe the breathing pattern in the dog and cat with pathology in the anatomic locations listed in the box.

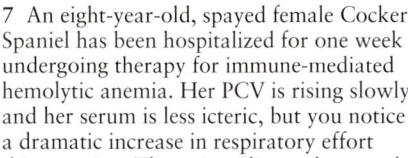

a. Large airway disease
b. Pharynx or larynx
c. Intrathoracic trachea
d. Pleural space disease (primarily air)
e. Parenchymal disease
f. Diaphragm
g. Small airway disease

7 & 8: Answers

7 i. There is enlargement of the pulmonary artery segment, a decrease in the size of the pulmonary vasculature and alveolar infiltrates in the left lung lobes, most visible on the ventrodorsal view.
ii. The relatively mild radiographic changes and normal $PaCO_2$ in conjunction with a significant hypoxemia and respiratory distress are suggestive of pulmonary thromboembolism.
iii. Pulmonary angiography or ventilation/perfusion scans can be performed to delineate the pulmonary parenchyma that is not perfused. Because these procedures are expensive and not widely available, treatment is usually initiated based on clinical signs, historical suspicion and blood-gas analysis.
iv. Oxygen supplementation, rest and treatment of the underlying disease process are the basic means of therapy. Heparin (200 units/kg i/v bolus, then 100–200 units/kg s/c qid) and warfarin therapy (0.05–1.0 mg/kg p/o sid) may prevent additional thromboemboli from forming. If the embolism had developed secondary to heartworm disease, steroids would also be indicated (prednisolone sodium succinate – 22mg/kg i/v). The use of thrombolytic agents are other options, but because of the risk of hemorrhage and the lack of clinical studies to support their use, these agents should be reserved for patients with life-threatening respiratory compromise

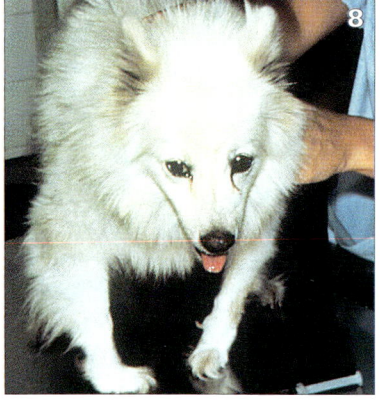

8 i. Increase in RR; change in breathing pattern; change in body posture (dog: will stand more, act restless, and arch back and abduct elbows (8); cat: does not change posture until very late); change in respiratory effort (cat breathes with abdomen very early, showing little intercostal muscle motion; dog breathes with intercostal muscles early and then with the abdomen); open mouth, neck extended breathing (dog more than cat); cyanosis; death.
ii. a – loud breathing heard without the aid of a stethescope; b – inspiratory stridor; c – expiratory stridor; d – dog: early – rapid shallow breathing; late – choppy breathing with the chest and abdomen moving in opposite directions, lung sound distant or muffled on auscultation; cat: early – no obvious signs; late – choppy breathing with the chest and abdomen moving in opposite directions, lung sounds can typically be heard throughout the thorax; tension pneumothorax dog and cat: barrel chested, little thoracic motion, strong, choppy breathing with diaphragmatic push on expiration, severe shock, and barely auscultable lungs; e – dog: smooth breathing with exaggerated inspiration and expiration of equal proportion; cat: smooth, rapid breathing with movement of the cupula (examine the thoracic inlet area closely for motion of the membrane – the abdomen moves in unison with the chest; f – dog: the abdomen moves inward with inspiration, rapid shallow movement of the chest, and strong diaphragmatic push on expiration; g – cat: short inspiration, prolonged expiration with a push of the diaphragm on expiration (high pitch wheezes heard, especially on expiration).

9–11: Questions

9 A dog presents with significant swelling of the lateral aspect of the thigh after having been shot (9). During resuscitation this area is noted to be expanding. A comminuted fracture of the femur is noted on radiographs.
i. What are the two most likely causes of the expanding hematoma?
ii. Could this patient suffer sufficient blood loss into this area to die?
iii. As the hematoma expands, what is the biggest concern?

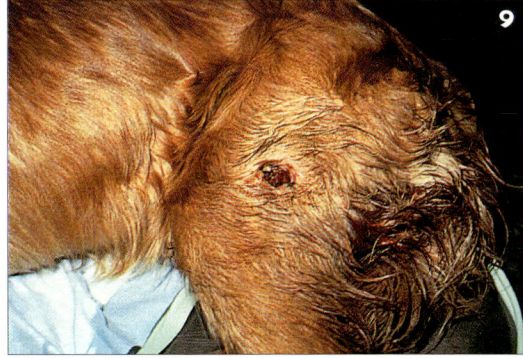

iv. What is the worst complication of this syndrome, and how will it need to be treated?
v. Immediate orthopedic surgery is not possible, yet pressure must be relieved due to concerns for vascular compromise to the area. What should be done?

10 This seven-month-old Doberman Pinscher is referred to your emergency clinic for evaluation of persistent hemorrhage following ovariohysterectomy. You suspect that the dog has von Willebrand's disease (VWD).
i. What diagnostic tests would you perform to confirm your suspicions?
ii. How would you treat this dog?

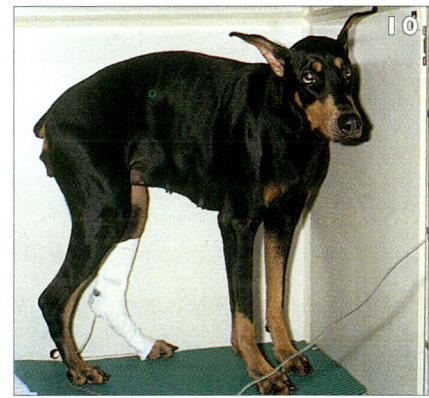

11 An owner calls about a ten-year-old, male castrated free-roaming cat that has an enlarged right eye that seems to fall out of the orbit.
i. What advice do you give the owner prior to transport?
At presentation, the cat has lacerations on the head and its claws are shredded. It is assumed that there was trauma. There is a prolapse of the right eye, no apparent laceration of the cornea, no rupture of the sclera, and a slight hyphema.
ii. How would you evaluate the eye prior to correction of the proptosis?
iii. How would you treat the proptosis?

9–11: Answers

9 i. Bleeding from torn muscles, periosteum and bone, and bleeding from a lacerated vessel secondary to bone fragments.
ii. Yes.
iii. Osseofascial compartment syndrome which is defined as an elevated interstitial pressure within a space defined and limited by a fascial envelope. This increase in pressure leads to decreased local blood flow and tissue hypoxia.
iv. If severe enough, compartment syndrome can cause temporary or permanent ischemia to the affected area. If permanent, limb amputation may be necessary.
v. The skin and underlying fascia should be incised and left open to allow continued expansion. The incision needs to be carried along the entire length of the compartment to allow full decompression. Any major vessels found to be bleeding should be ligated. The bone fragments may cause further trauma to muscle, vessels and nerves, and the limb should be stabilized in a padded spica bandage. Care should be taken to ensure the bandage does not restrict expansion of the muscle causing the compartment syndrome.

10 i. Platelet count, peripheral blood smear evaluation, PCV and ACT should be performed as initial screening tests. In a patient with VWD these tests would be within normal limits, as would PTT and PT. An abnormally prolonged buccal bleeding time is consistent with VWD. Confirmation of VWD is dependent on documenting abnormally low levels of factor VIII-related antigen.
ii. Coagulopathies associated with VWD should be treated in a similar way to other cases of hemorrhage. Fresh whole blood transfusion will provide RBCs as well as active coagulation factors. Fresh frozen plasma can be administered for coagulation factors. Adminstration of desmopressin acetate (DDAVP) to the donor (0.01% solution – 1 µg/kg s/c) 20–30 minutes before drawing the blood will cause massive release of VWF from endothelial stores, allowing transfusion of VWF-rich blood. DDAVP can also be administered directly to the patient with VWD, keeping in mind that the maximum protective effects of DDAVP last only 2–3 hours. Acepromazine should not be administered to the donor if platelet function is desired in the fresh blood.

11 i. The eye should be kept moist. If tolerated by the animal, sterile artificial tears or sterile water soluble lubricant is placed on the prolapsed globe. The animal is immediately transported while carefully restrained to prevent trauma to the eye.
ii. The pupil should be examined for response to light. In addition, the cornea is stained for evidence of ulceration.
iii. The animal must first be stabilized and any evidence of perfusion abnormalities corrected prior to general anesthesia for correction of the eye prolapse. Stain the cornea with fluorescein. Flush and lubricate the eye. Close the eyelids over the prolapsed globe – suture with mattress sutures and stints. If the eyelids cannot be closed over the eye, a canthotomy is required. Use antibiotic ointment.

12–14: Questions

12 This blood slide (**12**) was from a five-year-old, spayed female Miniature Poodle, presenting with a PCV of 10% and TS of 8.0 g/dl. She was depressed with tachypnea (RR – 40 bpm), tachycardia (HR – 180 bpm) with weak peripheral pulses, hypothermia (temperature – 98.96°F (37.2°C) and a prolonged CRT (>3 seconds) with icteric mucous membranes.
i. What is the most likely diagnosis?
ii. Why is this patient at risk of developing SIRS?
iii. Outline five points of treatment aimed at the prevention/treatment of SIRS in this patient.

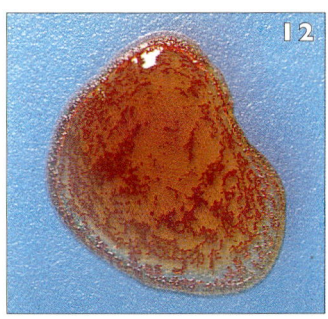

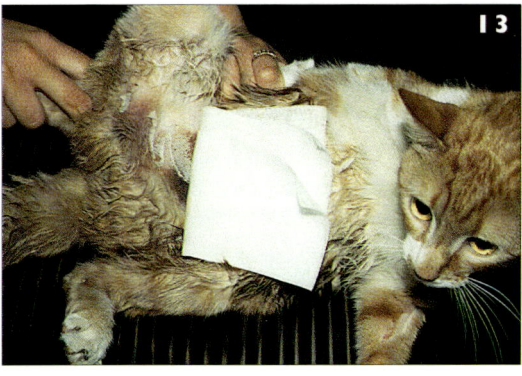

13 A two-year-old, castrated male, outdoor mixed-breed cat presented because he would posture to urinate and could not pass urine. The owners reported that the cat had vomited yellow foam twice in the last 2 hours. He had not eaten since he fell from the top of the refrigerator (12 hours ago). Physical examination revealed gray mucous membranes, temperature 97.88°F (36.6°C), weak femoral pulses and HR 140 bpm. The cat was estimated to be 8% dehydrated. There was a large subcutaneous hematoma throughout the inguinal and perineal area. (**13**). Urethral catheterization was unsuccessful. The urinary bladder was palpable, approximately half full with fluid. Radiographic examination of the abdomen found good contrast and a fluid-filled urinary bladder. Initial blood tests found: BUN – 120 mg/dl; creatinine – 8.0 mg/dl (707.2 µmol/l); K^+ – 8.0 mEq/l; Na^+ – 145 mEq/l. Venous blood gas: pH – 7.15; HCO_3 – 12 mEq/l; $PvCO_2$ – 45 mmHg.
i. What is the most likely diagnosis?
ii. What other diagnostic tests are indicated once the cat is stabilized?
iii. What is your plan for emergency stabilization?

14 A four-year-old, male, slightly obese Doberman Pinscher presents to the emergency clinic with an acute non-weightbearing lameness of the right hindlimb after a walk in the park. Physical examination is within normal limits. The dog is painful on palpation of the stifle joint and the stifle seems to be swollen. Further examination is impossible (aggressive dog).
i. What are your further diagnostic steps?
ii. Radiography of the stifle joint shows an increased size of the articular capsule; no obvious fractures can be seen. What are your differentials at this time?
iii. Examination under sedation is positive for a cranial drawer movement. What other test could be used to diagnose cranial cruciate ligament rupture?
iv. What is your treatment of choice?

12–14: Answers

12 i. Immune-mediated hemolytic anemia (IMHA).
ii. The patient is in a state of poor perfusion and hypoxemia which leads to peripheral tissue ischemia. Red cell destruction leads to microaggregates of red cell carcasses, inflammatory cells and platelets which can lead to secondary DIC and organ ischemia. Complement activation secondary to antigen-antibody reaction results in release of C3a and C5a, leading to smooth muscle contraction and neutrophil chemotaxis. The accumulation of the neutrophils and subsequent degranulation will cause further endothelial and cell membrane damage. Endothelial cell damage stimulates the coagulation cascade. Cell membrane damage leads to release of arachidonic acid metabolites.
iii.
• Restore peripheral perfusion – i/v fluid support.
• Oxygen supplementation.
• Replenish RBC mass if PCV drops rapidly below 15%.
• Treat the immune response with steroid therapy ± other immunosuppressive therapy.
• Consider subcutaneous heparin ± plasma for AT III.
• Monitor closely for the development of DIC and thromboembolic phenomenon, utilizing coagulation panels, ACT, platelet counts, AT III.

13 i. Inability to urinate, unsuccessful catheterization of a urinary bladder with urine retained, severe azotemia, hyperkalemia and metabolic acidosis suggest post-renal urinary tract obstruction or rupture. Unsuccessful urethral catheterization and inguinal and perineal hematomas suggest urethral blockage or rupture rather than ruptured urinary bladder.
ii. A contrast retrograde urethrogram with water soluble contrast media would outline a urethral stricture, rupture or blockage. If this does not reveal an abnormality, an IVP would highlight the urinary tract bilaterally. An ultrasound would direct further investigation into the kidneys, urinary bladder and other abdominal organs.
iii. Initial stabilization should address the intravascular and interstitial volume deficits. A combination of crystalloids and colloids should be administered until perfusion and hydration are restored. An ECG should be done. If significant arrhythmias are present, due to raised K^+, and associated with poor perfusion, immediate stabilization of the arrhythmias is obtained with 0.2 units/kg regular insulin followed by 2 grams glucose per unit of insulin. Urinary flow can be restored on a temporary basis by placing a catheter into the urinary bladder percutaneously. Assessment of the skin hematoma and evaluation of the cat's coagulation profile is required. The radiographs are assessed for pelvic injuries. Urine output and CVP are monitored. Prepare for surgical repair of the urethra.

14 i. Sedation with analgesia, repeat orthopedic examination, radiographs (area depending on orthopedic examination).
ii. Cranial cruciate ligament rupture, traumatic contusion, arthritis of different origins, patellar luxations.
iii. Tibial compression.
iv. Arthrotomy, debridement and stabilization of the joint.

15–17: Questions

15 A 12-year-old, spayed female domestic shorthair cat was presented after a fire in the apartment (15). The cat was found hiding under the bed and was presented very shortly afterwards.
i. What problems do you anticipate?
ii. The cat is collapsed with pale mucous membranes and severe respiratory distress both on inspiration and expiration. Why does the cat have pale mucous membranes?
iii. How will you treat this animal (list in order of priority)?

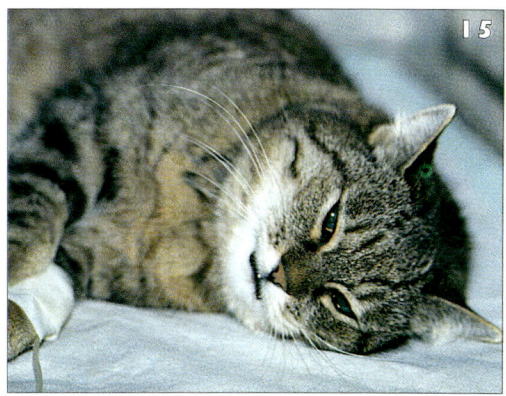

16 This two-year-old mixed-breed bitch had four puppies 16 days ago. The puppies seem healthy but the owners report that the dam is salivating, walking stiffly, panting and has muscle tremors.
i. What is your tentative diagnosis?
ii. What potential problems in the dam should be ruled out with your initial data base and physical examination?
iii. What is your management plan for this case?
iv. What problems have been associated with oral and parenteral calcium administration?

17 i. Match as many of the numbers as are appropriate with each antibiotic:

a. First generation cephalosporin	1. Bactericidal
b. Metronidazole	2. Bacteristatic
c. Gentamicin	3. Gram-negative spectrum
d. Amoxicillin	4. Gram-positive spectrum
e. Trimethoprim-sulfa	5. Anaerobic spectrum
f. Enrofloxacin	6. Penetrates the intact blood brain
g. Chloramphenicol	barrier to therapeutic levels
h. Tetracycline	
i. Clindamycin	

ii. What is a nosocomial infection, and what is the most common source of this infection?
iii. Provide methods for minimizing nosocomial infections.
iv. Provide a method for monitoring for nosocomial infections.

15–17: Answers

15 i. Thermal burns, respiratory distress, pneumonia, shock, dehydration.
ii. The pale mucous membranes reflect poor perfusion. Carbon monoxide would show bright red mucous membranes.
iii. Use aseptic techniques; supplemental oxygen; obtain a patent airway (suction or tracheotomy if required – culture airway if invasive intervention required); positive pressure ventilation, if required, with 100% oxygen; i/v catheter and crystalloid therapy; large molecular weight colloid to minimize crystalloid requirements; clip the fur and look for burns; wound care – with culture – topical; bacteriocidal antibiotics as indicated; analgesic sedation.

16 i. Eclampsia.
ii. Hypocalcemia is often accompanied by hyperthermia, dehydration, hypoglycemia and cardiac arrhythmias.
iii. Ten percent calcium gluconate (0.5–1.5 ml/kg) should be administered slowly i/v until clinical signs regress. The drug must be discontinued if bradycardia or other arrhythmias are noted on ECG. Vomition or 'licking the lips' are indications that i/v administration should be discontinued. A second dose of calcium gluconate (1–2 ml/kg) can be given s/c if it is diluted 50:50 with saline. Fever, dehydration and hypoglycemia can be managed with i/v fluid therapy. Ideally, the pups should be removed and hand raised, but if they are allowed to remain with the dam, she should receive oral calcium supplementation (25–50 mg/kg/day divided every 8 hours) until lactation is completed.
iv. Calcium supplementation prior to whelping inhibits parathormone secretion and makes the dam more prone to hypocalcemia during lactation. If i/v calcium is administered too rapidly, cardiac arrhythmias may result. Oversupplementation with calcium may cause arrhythmias, neurologic impairment, GI dysfunction and renal failure. Calcium chloride must never be administered i/m or s/c, as tissue necrosis and skin sloughs can occur.

17 i. a – 1, 3, 4, 5; b – 1, 5, 6; c – 1, 3, (some 4); d – 1, 3, 4, 5, 6 if inflamed; e – 1, 3, 4, ±5, 6 (when inflamed); f – 1, 3, ±4, 6 (very low levels only); g – 2, (can be 1 at higher concentrations), 3, 4, 5, 6; h – 2, some 3, 4, 5; i – 1 (depending on concentration), 2, 4, 5, 6 (if meninges inflamed).
ii. One that is acquired from the hospital. These bacteria are frequently very antibiotic-resistant. The most common source is the hands of personnel.
iii. Ensuring good hygiene with the doctor and nursing staff is of utmost importance. Just wearing latex gloves does not prevent passage of bacteria. Personnel must wash carefully between patients with a bactericidal soap. In addition, thoroughly cleaning and disinfecting the environment is crucial. The junction where a tube or catheter invades the body should be cleaned, covered and monitored for contamination. Establishing an antibiotic protocol is critical. The hospital should choose two or three antibiotics that are first choice, selected prior to culture and sensitivity results are returned. The common use of these antibiotics then limits the bacteria in the environment to becoming resistant to these alone. Should a wide variety of potent antibiotics be used commonly, then a population of environmental bacteria will grow with a very wide antibiotic resistance, making treatment potentially unsuccessful.
iv. The bacterial culture and sensitivity results from catheters and equipment should be monitored for evidence of resistance to the hospital's first choice antibiotics. Should this be occurring frequently, then a thorough cleaning and disinfection of the environment is warranted. In addition, careful scrutiny of personal hygiene is necessary. Invasive equipment such as endotracheal tubes, catheters, ventilators, etc, should be cultured occasionally and their antibiotic resistance patterns examined if contamination found.

18 & 19: Questions

18 This four-month-old, male Newfoundland puppy had epistaxis for several days (**18**). The dog has hemophilia and received two blood transfusions 1 month previously for the same problem. The dog was given another blood transfusion because of significant anemia and bleeding. During the transfusion the dog became lethargic, developed a fever, vomited several times and shivered.

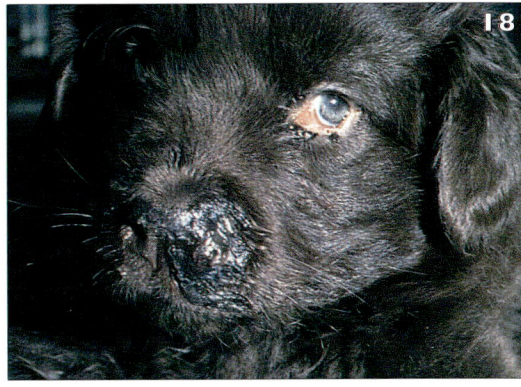

i. What complications have to be considered?
ii. Which types of hypersensitivity reactions play a role?
iii. What is the treatment?
iv. How can these complications be avoided?

19 A seven-month-old, female Toy Poodle (**19a**) jumped from a footstool onto the floor, yelped and became reluctant to move. The dog is ambulatory, but conscious proprioceptive deficits are noted on all four limbs. Pain is easily elicited upon cervical palpation. Cervical radiographs (**19b**) are taken with the dog under anesthesia.

i. What is the diagnosis?
ii. Congenital absence of what structure predisposes to this situation?
iii. What non-surgical therapy could be used to treat this patient?
iv. What are the limitations of using this non-surgical treatment as the definitive therapy?
v. Describe a surgical treatment performed from a ventral cervical approach.

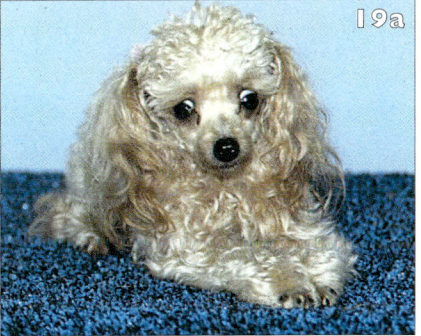

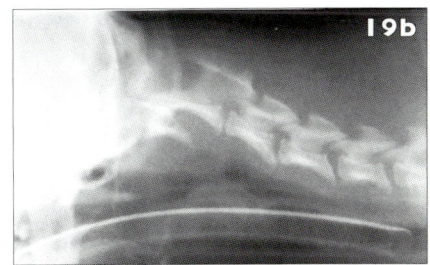

18 & 19: Answers

18 i. Lethargy, fever and vomiting can be the result of hypersensitivity reactions to donor WBCs and foreign antigens in the donor blood. Acute intravascular hemolysis and sepsis can result from contaminated blood. Shivering can be due to the fever but can also be caused by hypocalcemia as a result of citrate toxicity.
ii. Type I hypersentivitiy reactions against donor white cells, foreign proteins or other foreign material. Type II or IV (delayed) reactions can occur against the transfused RBCs.
iii. Stop the transfusion immediately. Start shock therapy. If early in the reaction, antihistamines may be of benefit. Glucocorticoids can decrease the host's immune response. Check for hemolysis and hypocalcemia. Check for transfusion contamination, and monitor for DIC and kidney failure.
iv. Transfusion reactions are minimized by administering only A-negative blood that has been cross-matched to the recipient. The blood must be handled properly during collection and administration. The transfusion is given slowly (3–4 hours) if time permits. The use of components will minimize exposure to donor WBCs, proteins and other foreign material. Cryoprecipitate or fresh frozen plasma avoids the risk of hemolysis if the patient is not significantly anemic. The patient is monitored closely for transfusion reaction.

19 i. Atlantoaxial instability/luxation.
ii. Absence of the dens.
iii. Neck brace, cage rest (at least 3 weeks) and analgesics.
iv. Conservative management relies on scar tissue for stabilization; therefore, minimal trauma could result in recurrence of atlantoaxial luxation and associated clinical signs.
v. Transarticular atlantoaxial pins.

20 & 21: Questions

20 This two-year-old, male Irish Setter (33 kg) was hit by a car 1 hour prior to presentation (**20**). The dog was able to walk on three limbs. The dog is fully vaccinated, has had no food within the last 6 hours and the owner has not noticed any urination since the accident. The dog is depressed but responsive to its environment. Physical examination: temperature – 101.3°F (38.5°C); HR – 160 bpm; RR – 40 bpm; bilateral lung sounds present – the left-sided thoracic auscultation reveals slightly harsher lung sounds compared to the right side.

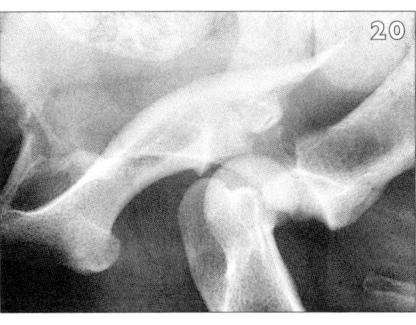

Abdominal palpation is non-painful, no fluid wave can be detected, gut sounds are present and the urinary bladder cannot be palpated. The dog is non-weightbearing lame on the left hindlimb, painful on palpation of the lateral proximal femoral region, and deep palpation of the bones of the hindlimbs is not possible without sedation.
i. Summarize the initial resuscitation.
ii. What further diagnostic steps would you take to assess the dog's injuries?
iii. What is the radiographic finding?
iv. What is the best treatment?
v. What are possible complications with this injury?
vi. What further radiographic studies can be done to rule out urinary tract trauma?

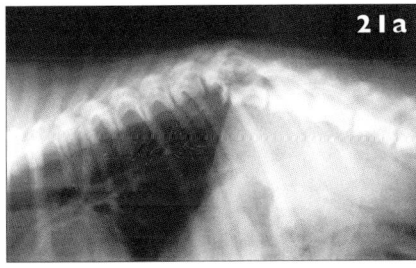
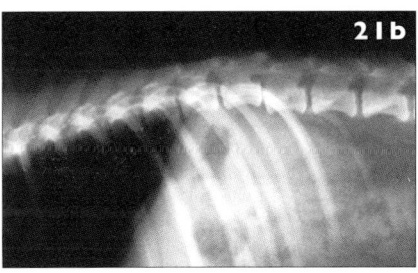

21 Lateral spinal radiographs were taken of two different dogs (**21a**, **21b**) that were struck by automobiles.
i. Describe the spinal injuries in both of these dogs. (Assume 13 ribs bilaterally.)
ii. Based on these radiographs, which dog can be assumed to have spinal cord transection?
iii. On what could you base your prognosis in the other dog?
iv. The dog without radiographic evidence of spinal cord transection is presented to you within 30 minutes of being struck by an automobile. There is questionable voluntary motor movement but deep pain is present. What corticosteroid could be used as part of your treatment for the spinal cord injury, and what is the treatment protocol for its use?
v. Why is i/v fluid therapy begun prior to administration of i/v corticosteroids?
vi. Why might the dog with spinal cord transection have extensor rigidity in the forelimbs? What is the name given to this syndrome?

20 & 21: Answers

20 i. Oxygen by nasal catheter, flow-by or oxygen hood; i/v fluid resuscitation with crystalloid fluid solution (Plasma-Lyte, lactated Ringer's solution) and colloids, continuous monitoring of HR, RR, mucous membrane color, BP and lung sounds; analgesia with opioids.
ii. Thoracic radiographs to rule out pneumothorax, pulmonary contusion and thoracic effusion. Abdominal radiographs to evaluate for intra-abdominal injuries including the integrity of the genitourinary system. Initial laboratory evaluation of PCV, TS, BUN, glucose and electrolytes. Survey radiographs of the left femur including the pelvis.
iii. Cranial acetabular fracture with severe displacement.
iv. Open reduction and internal fixation with a bone plate, screws and orthopedic wire.
v. Osteoarthritis even after optimal reduction; trauma or iatrogenic-induced sciatic nerve injury; intrapelvic soft tissue trauma including the intestinal tract or the genitourinary tract.
vi. After rehydration of the dog, an excretory urogram to detect renal and ureteral trauma. A positive contrast cystogram is performed to rule out a bladder tear, and a retrograde urethrogram can be used to confirm urethral damage.

21 i. A fracture of T11 with 100% displacement of the spinal canal in **21a**; a luxation of T12–T13 with minimal displacement is seen in **21b**.
ii. The dog with the T11 fracture with 100% displacement.
iii. Neurologic examination, particularly the presence or absence of deep pain.
iv. Methylprednisolone sodium succinate. The treatment protocol consists of the following i/v doses: 30 mg/kg initially, then 15 mg/kg at 2 and 6 hours, then 2.5 mg/kg/hour CRI for the next 42 hours.
v. I/v administration of corticosteroids can cause hypotension, and the patient is usually traumatized and prone to shock.
vi. Transection of ascending inhibitory innervation from the lumbar spinal cord removes inhibition of motor nerves of the thoracic limbs, and extensor reflexes predominate. This is the Schiff-Sherrington Syndrome.

22–24: Questions

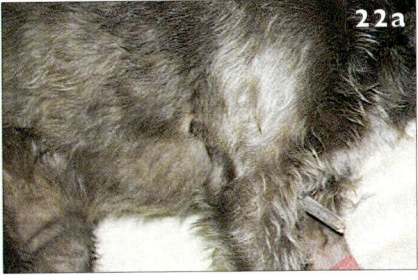
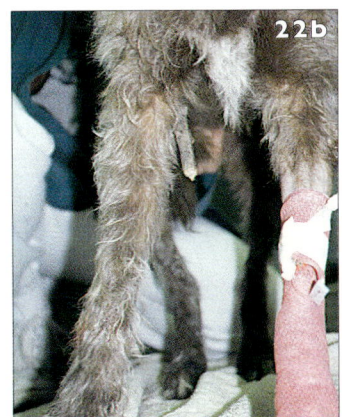

22 A seven-year-old mixed-breed dog walked home after having been in the woods. On presentation the dog is quiet and alert, has a HR of 140 bpm and a RR of 36 bpm (**22a, 22b**).
i. What is your initial plan for evaluation and stabilization?
ii. What is the treatment of choice in this situation?

23 i. List the four sources of input to the medullary vomiting center.
ii. What is the role of anticholinergic drugs in the treatment of gastrointestinal disease?
iii. True or false: pharmacological intervention is indicated for all vomiting patients. If false, state when it is indicated.
iv. Name a side-effect of chlorpromazine that may limit its use in the critically ill patient.
v. The appearance of vomitus can often help to define the abnormal portion of the GI tract. Match each of the following color descriptions of vomitus with the anatomic source (more than one answer may be correct):
1. Blood   a. Gastric
2. White, mucoid   b. Biliary reflux
3. Fetid, green/brown   c. Duodenal
4. Yellow/green   d. Esophageal

24 A dog is presented with diarrhea. The owner also reports the dog is defecating frequently and with tenesmus.
i. These findings suggest the problem is in which segment of the GI tract?
ii. Label each of the following characteristics as suggestive of either large (LB) or small bowel (SB) disease:
a. Presence of excess mucus.
b. Melena.
c. Increased fecal volume.
d. Tenesmus.
e. Significant weight loss.
f. Hematochezia.
iii. List the four pathologic mechanisms of diarrhea. For which mechanism(s) are antidiarrheal drugs not indicated?

22–24: Answers

22 i. The dog should be treated initially for shock with i/v fluids. Thoracic radiographs may reveal the presence of a pneumothorax or hemothorax which would be evidence that the stick had penetrated through the thoracic wall. The stick will not be radiopaque, therefore absence of free air or blood in the thorax does not rule out the possibility of penetration. Before manipulating the dog for radiographs, consider cutting the stick closer to the skin surface to minimize the risk of iatrogenic trauma.
ii. If the dog appears stable, it is best to remove the foreign object under conditions for sterile surgery. The dog is intubated to facilitate mechanical ventilation and the thorax is prepared for surgery. Premature removal of the stick may result in the rapid development of pneumothorax or hemothorax and hypovolemic shock. Surgical exploration of the route of the stick provides the opportunity to visualize the structures along it, and to evaluate and repair any damaged tissues. In this case, a thoracotomy was necessary because the stick had passed along the medial aspect of the thoracic wall and punctured the right crus of the diaphragm without injuring lung lobes. Tube thoracostomy to permit drainage and broad-spectrum antibiotics are indicated after surgery.

23 i. Peripheral sensory receptors; chemoreceptor trigger zone; higher CNS centers; vestibular system.
ii. There are few if any indications for their use. They are not antiemetic; they reduce motility which is often already reduced by the primary disease process. The development of ileus predisposes the patient to bacterial translocation and to aspiration pneumonia.
iii. False; antiemetics are indicated when the physical demands of vomiting are detrimental to the patient (exhaustion, increased intracranial pressure, decreased gag reflex causing increased risk of aspiration) or when fluid, electrolyte and acid–base abnormalities cannot be corrected because of continued losses.
iv. Hypotension, especially in the volume depleted patient.
v. 1 – d, a, c; 2 – a, d; 3 – c; 4 – b.

24 i. Large bowel.
ii. a – LB; b – SB; c – SB; d – LB; e – SB; f – LB.
iii. Osmotic (decreased absorption); secretory; exudative (increased mucosal permeability); altered motility. Antimotility drugs are not indicated and may be contraindicated in conditions where increased contact time between luminal contents and a damaged mucosa may promote absorption of organisms or toxins.

25 & 26: Questions

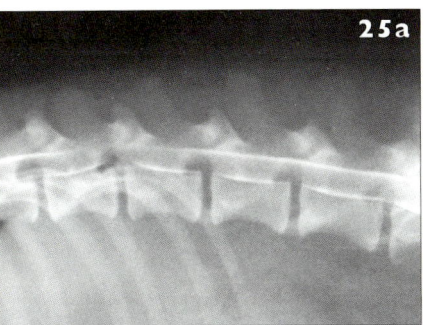
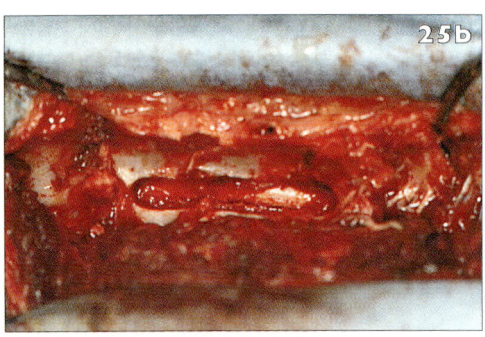

25 A six-year-old Dachshund is presented with acute (less than 6 hours since the onset of clinical signs) group IV-A thoracolumbar intervertebral disc disease. A myelogram (**25a**) has been performed, followed by decompressive surgery (**25b**, **25c**) (in **25c** the forceps are pointing to extruded disc material in the ventral aspect of the spinal canal).
i. Where is the lesion based on this myelogram? (Assume 13 ribs bilaterally.)
ii. Would you expect that this dog had hyperreflexia or hyporeflexia of the patellar reflex?
iii. What peripheral nerve is tested by the patellar reflex?
iv. What decompressive surgical procedure has been performed?
v. The decision as to which side to perform this procedure is based on what factors?
vi. Give at least two advantages and one disadvantage to this surgical procedure as compared to a dorsal laminectomy.
vii. What initial neurologic examination finding indicates performing a durotomy?

26 A three-year-old, castrated male gray cat was presented for a 2-week history of anorexia. Physical examination found the cat to be obese, though the owner has reported a 1.5 kg weight loss. The cat has significant icterus. Temperature – 100.94°F (38.3°C); HR – 200 bpm; RR – 24 bpm; CRT – 2 seconds; mucous membranes – yellow/pink; enlarged liver palpated on abdominal examination. The pulses were strong and the chest auscultated normally. An abdominal ultrasound demonstrated the liver to have a hyperechogenic texture, similar to the echotexture of the falciform fat. A liver aspirate revealed hepatocytes filled with fat. There was no evidence of inflammation.
i. Identify the serum biochemical tests that demonstrate liver function.
ii. What is the most likely diagnosis for this cat, and what critical electrolyte disorders can be anticipated?
iii. Comment on the following therapeutic modalities for this cat: nutrition, carnitine, taurine, zinc, vitamin E, arginine, thiamine, vitamin K1.
iv. Care must be taken when giving diazepam to these cats. Why?
v. Adding glucose to this cat's fluids can make his problem worse. Why?

25 & 26: Answers

25 i. There is a compressive lesion at the T13–L1 intervertebral disc space.
ii. Hyperreflexia due to the location of the lesion.
iii. The femoral nerve.
iv. A hemilaminectomy has been performed to gain access to the spinal canal and decompress the spinal cord by removal of the extruded disc material.
v. Historical lateralization, i.e. the owner reports that the problem started with one side affected more than the other.
Lateralization of neurologic signs on the neurologic examination.
Myelographic lateralization.
Handedness of the surgeon (right-handed surgeon performs left-sided hemilaminectomy because of ease of dissection).
vi. Advantages include: the need to elevate musculature off bone on only one side of the spinal column; better access to the ventral part of the spinal canal; less chance of laminectomy membrane formation. A disadvantage is that access to both sides of the spinal canal cannot be achieved, therefore it may be difficult or impossible to retrieve extruded disc material if the wrong side is approached (such as when the lesion could not be lateralized preoperatively).
vii. Absence of deep pain would indicate performing a durotomy for prognostic purposes.

26 i. Bilirubin, if there is no hemolytic disease; glucose; albumin; PT and PTT; cholesterol; bile acids.
ii. Hepatic lipidosis. Significant hypokalemia causing muscle and myocardial weakness, and hypophosphatemia causing RBC hemolysis.
iii.
- *Nutrition.* These cats need 60–80 kcal/kg/day. A balanced feline maintenance food or liquid diet made for cats is ideal. If a human product is used, will need to supplement with arginine.
- *Carnitine.* This is necessary to export fatty acids into the hepatocyte for fat metabolism. Supplemented (l-carnitine) at 250–500 mg/day.
- *Taurine.* This is an essential amino acid in the cat and is excreted in the urine and bile salts. It is necessary for heart function and has some antioxidant function. A deficiency can lead to retinal degeneration and dilated cardiomyopathy. Supplemented at 250–500 mg/day.
- *Zinc.* Important for many enzyme functions and intermediary metabolic functions of the liver. Supplemented at 7–10 mg/kg/day as zinc acetate.
- *Vitamin E.* This is a natural antioxidant and is supplemented at 20–100 IU/day. Absorption from the GI tract may be impaired since it is a fat soluble vitamin.
- *Arginine.* This is an essential amino acid in the cat and must be supplemented if the diet is home-made or human. Supplemented at 1000 mg/day.
- *Thiamine.* This water soluble vitamin must be supplemented and is critical for brain energy production. Supplemented at 100 mg/day.
- *Vitamin K1.* Most of these cats have prolonged clotting times, but do not bleed. Vitamin K1 is given at 5 mg i/m every 12 hours for 2–3 doses.

iv. Diazepam is metabolized in the liver. With impaired liver function, the drug has a very prolonged effect in these cats.
v. I/v glucose can cause increased fat accumulation in the hepatocytes.

27–29: Questions

27 This blood is from a seven-year-old, intact female Labrador Retriever presented for evaluation of weakness (**27**). PCV – 9%; TS – 8.0 g/dl.
i. What test has been performed, and what is the abnormality pictured?
ii. What does this abnormality suggest about the etiology of this dog's anemia?
iii. Is a Coombs' test necessary to confirm the diagnosis?
iv. How would you treat this patient?

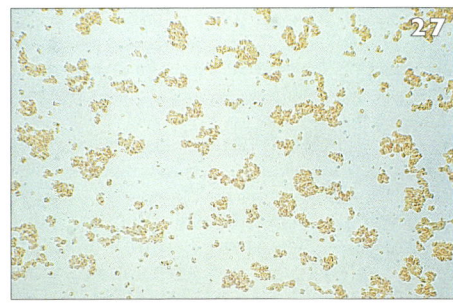

28 This domestic shorthair cat (5 kg) presented with a 3-day history of vomiting and anorexia (**28**). His HR is 140 bpm, and he has pale mucous membranes with a 2–3 sec CRT. Dehydration was assessed at 10% based on skin turgor and mucous membrane moisture.
i. In which fluid compartment is the deficit in this cat (intravascular, interstitial, intracellular, or a combination)? Justify your answer.
ii. What type of fluid would you choose to treat this patient, and why?
iii. Calculate the fluid amount and rate of administration for replacement of dehydration.

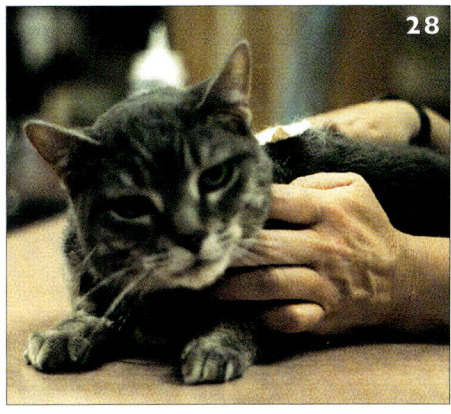

29 A ten-year-old, male German Shepherd Dog is evaluated for anorexia and weight loss over 1 week and acute onset profound lethargy/exercise intolerance. The dog is weak, has a temperature of 104°F (40°C) and is tachypneic with mild crackles ventrally and harsh lung sounds dorsally. A systolic and diastolic murmur is auscultated over the left heart base, though the owner reports a murmur had been noted since the dog was 4 months old.
i. What is your tentative diagnosis?

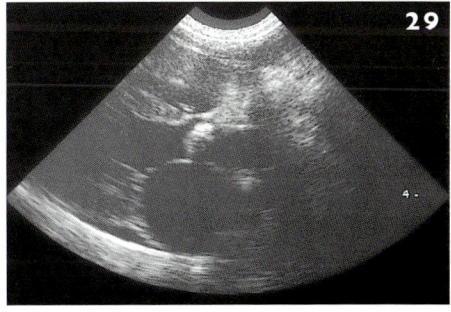

ii. What is the likely source of the murmur? What other valve(s) may be involved?
iii. Chest radiographs reveal a diffuse interstitial pattern and only mild cardiomegaly. An echocardiogram is performed (**29**). What is your diagnosis and how are the radiographic findings consistent with this diagnosis?
iv. What diagnostic test(s) would best confirm your suspicion?
v. What treatment would you initiate in the acute phase and what is the long-term prognosis?

27–29: Answers

27 i. Slide test for autoagglutination. Autoagglutination.
ii. The presence of autoagglutination, when differentiated from rouleaux formation, suggests that this patient's anemia is immune-mediated in origin.
iii. A positive result in saline slide agglutination negates the need to perform a Coombs' test.
iv. Treatment of IMHA depends on non-specific suppression of the immune system, with glucocorticoids being the mainstay of therapy. In dogs with autoagglutination, aggressive treatment with prednisone (2–4 mg/kg p/o bid) and a cytotoxic drug is warranted from the beginning. Cyclophosphamide (50 mg/m^2 p/o 4 days per week) or azathioprine (2 mg/kg p/o daily for 4 days, then every other day) may be used. Cyclosporin A (10 mg/kg p/o bid for 10 days) may be used in patients with intravascular hemolysis.

28 i. This cat has both an intravascular and an interstitial compartment fluid deficit. The pale gum color and prolonged CRT suggest poor perfusion related to hypovolemia. Skin turgor and mucous membrane moisture suggest dehydration, a fluid deficit in the interstitial space.
ii. An isotonic crystalloid for fluid replacement of the interstitial and intravascular space, or a combination of isotonic crystalloid and colloid, with the colloid remaining in the intravascular space.
iii. 500 ml (5 kg × 0.10 = 0.5 liters). In addition, the cat requires approximately 10 ml/hour maintenance fluid rate. This cat can tolerate a relatively quick hydration replacement rate as it appears to have been ill only 3 days. Therefore, replacing the fluid deficit over 10 hours (500 ml/10 hours = 50 ml/hour) while providing a maintenance rate would require an infusion of approximately 60 ml/hour for 10 hours. This fluid rate may need to be readjusted if further fluid loss in the form of vomiting or diarrhea occurs.

29 i. Bacterial endocarditis with secondary acute congestive heart failure or embolic pneumonia. Large breed, male dogs are affected with bacterial endocarditis more commonly. However, it is possible that the murmur is due to congenital aortic stenosis and an infection elsewhere, neoplasia, or because immune-mediated disease is present.
ii. The origin of the murmur is most likely the aortic valve. Typically, a decrescendo diastolic murmur from aortic insufficiency is present and is usually loudest in early diastole. A systolic murmur may or may not be present; in fact, there may be no murmur at all. The mitral valve in dogs is affected most commonly in bacterial endocarditis, then the aortic valve.
iii. When acute mitral regurgitation or aortic insufficiency occurs secondary to bacterial endocarditis, the increased left ventricular volume rapidly increases left ventricular end-diastolic pressure due to limits imposed by the myocardium and pericardial sac; thus, pulmonary edema develops with only mild to moderate compensatory cardiomegaly. The left atrium is usually normal in size as at the time of diagnosis.
iv. Serial blood cultures should be drawn. Positive blood cultures have been obtained in 88% of affected dogs when more than one sample was drawn.
v. Diuretics and vasodilators (hydralazine or angiotensin-converting enzyme inhibitor) should be initiated to control the edema, reduce valvular regurgitation and improve forward cardiac output. Myocardial contractility usually remains within normal limits until late in the disease process. A broad-spectrum antibiotic (cephalosporin or penicillin) in combination with an aminoglycoside are started until culture results are available. Corticosteroids are contraindicated.

30–32: Questions

30 A 30 kg, six-year-old, spayed female Labrador presents after being hit by a car (**30**). Primary survey reveals the patient has rapid shallow breathing with poor perfusion. Pulmonary auscultation reveals an absence of lung sounds over the entire left thorax with decreased lung sounds on the right. After multiple thoracocentesis positive for air, the decision is made to place a thoracostomy tube.
i. Describe the process of thoracostomy tube placement, including the approximate size

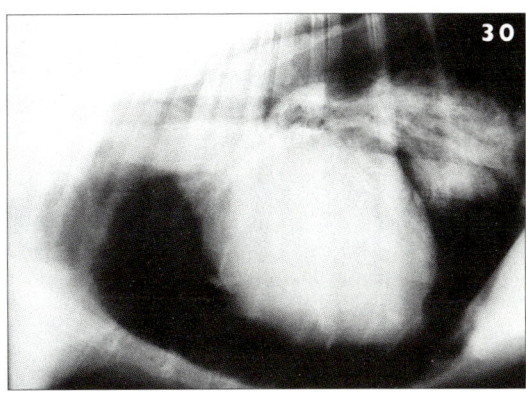

of the chest tube, the location of insertion and the positioning relative to the problem.
ii. What are the potential complications during tube placement and maintenance?
iii. What are the different methods of suctioning?
iv. How is the decision made to remove the thorocostomy tube?

31 A four-year-old, castrated male Laborador Retriever presented 2 days after suffering blunt trauma to his lateral thoracic wall (**31**). He had developed a firm, painful, red, expanding swelling of the skin and subcutaneous tissues at the area of trauma. On presentation, temperature was 104°F (40.0°C) and HR was 130 bpm.
i. What is the most likely diagnosis?
ii. Surgical resection of the involved tissue was performed. What specific concerns should be addressed during wound repair?
iii. What are the antibiotic(s) of choice in this patient?

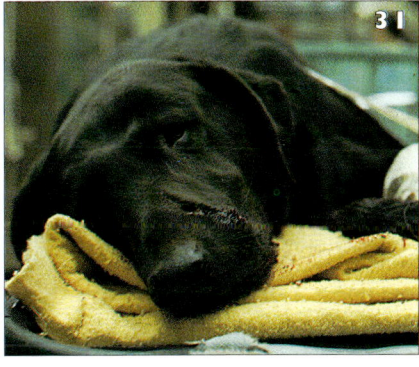

32 Two cats present simultaneously. One has urethral obstruction of unknown duration; HR – 60 bpm; temperature – 99.5°F (37.5°C); RR – 8 bpm; CRT – 2–3 seconds; mucous membranes – pale pink, dry; severe mental depression; PCV – 50%; TS – 8.0 g/dl. The other cat is anemic; HR – 240 bpm; temperature – 104°F (40°C); RR – 36 bpm; CRT – 1–2 seconds; mucous membranes – pale, moist; mentally alert; PCV – 10%; TS – 6.5 g/dl.
i. How would you prioritize these two animals?
ii. What is your immediate management of the most critical cat?
iii. As you work on the most critical patient, what instructions would you give to begin treating the other cat?

30–32: Answers

30 i. The thoracostomy tube should be placed on the side that is most affected; however, some patients require bilateral thoracostomy tubing. The lateral thorax is surgically prepared from the caudal edge of the scapula to the mid-abdomen. The skin of the thorax is pulled cranially by an assistant. A local anesthetic block is placed at the insertion site (skin to pleura) as well as an intercostal block. A small incision is made between the ribs at the level of the 7th or 8th mid-dorsal intercostal space and a hemostat is used to perforate the pleura and assist in introducing the tube. The thoracostomy tube should be approximately the size of the main stem bronchus and have 3–5 holes in the end. The tube is inserted with the aid of a stylet into the cranial thorax to the level of the 2nd–3rd rib. The stylet is removed and the tube twisted along its axis to make sure it is in the cranial thorax. The skin is released and allowed to form a tunnel over the tube. All holes are within the pleural cavity and not in the subcutaneous tissue. The tube is fixed to the rib periosteum on both the dorsal and ventral side of the tube. A second fixation ligature is placed several centimeters from the exit site. A sterile dressing is then placed.
ii. Include lung trauma, air leak and infection.
iii. Constant low negative pressure evacuation via underwater suction has the advantage of aiding in control of hemorrhages and sealing of pleuropulmonary leaks by keeping the pleural surfaces in contact.
Intermittent, gentle hand suctioning is adequate when air leaks are not life-threatening, and it allows quantitation of air and fluid.
A Heimlich valve.
iv. They are removed when they are no longer productive. When the amount of air removed has become minimal (1–2 ml of air/kg/suction) the tube is clamped for 12–24 hours without suctioning. 2–4 ml/kg/day of sterile fluid production can be expected just from the presence of the tube.

31 i. Cellulitis/fasciitis, with possible development of SIRS.
ii. Full exploration and resection of inflamed tissue; culture (aerobic and anaerobic) of involved tissue; adequate drainage; mark around the wound; compression bandage. Be prepared to enter the chest if required during exploration of the wound.
iii. Broad-spectrum antibiotics to cover aerobic and anaerobic bacteria, e.g. first generation cephalosporin and metronidazole.

32 i. The first cat has a life-threatening bradycardia and is treated first.
ii. I/v catheter, blood for prefluid electrolytes and renal tests, i/v fluids, ECG monitoring, administer 1 unit regular insulin with 2 grams glucose, urethral catheterization and closed urinary collection system.
iii. Prepare for i/v catheter, oxygen, blood tests, blood smear, FeLV testing, CBC and reticulocyte count; prepare for blood transfusion if indicated.

33 & 34: Questions

33 A four-year-old Sealyham Terrier presented with acute onset unilateral (right) ocular pain. There was marked blepharospasm and excessive lacrimation. Initial examination revealed episcleral congestion and mild corneal edema (**33**). The pupil was semidilated and non-responsive to light. The iris was bowed posteriorly but the fundus appeared normal, although the dog was blind on this side.
i. Describe the pathology seen in the eye.
ii. What is your diagnosis?
iii. Why is the dog blind in this eye?
iv. What treatment would you prescribe?

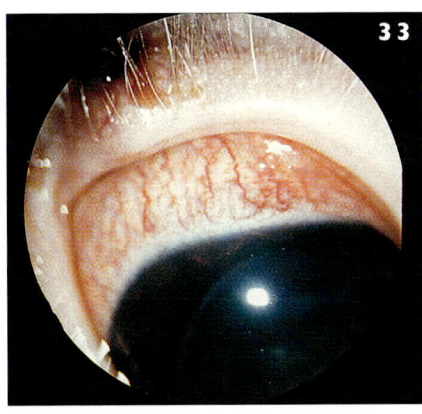

34 A ten-month-old, spayed female English Sheepdog is presented with the complaint of polyuria/polydipsia for the previous 2 days and vomiting several times this morning (**34a**). The dog was spayed with no complications at 6 months of age. Presently she is being treated with vitamin K1 for a confirmed rodenticide ingestion 5 days ago. Important physical examination findings include: HR – 70 bpm; CRT – 4 seconds; estimated 5% dehydration; weak femoral pulses; rectal temperature – 99°F (37.2°C).
i. Which of the following should be included in the differential diagnosis – a. lead poisoning; b. endocrinopathy; c. cystitis; d. allergic reaction; e. neuropathy?
  Initial diagnostic results: BP – 85/60 mmHg (11.3/8.0 kPa); PCV – 58%; TS – 7.1 g/dl; Na^+ – 110 mEq/l; K^+ – 7.1 mEq/l; chloride – 116 mEq/l; urine SG – 1.017, no cells on sediment; BUN labstick – 50–80 mg/dl; ethylene glycol test – negative; glucose – 60 mg/dl (3.36 mmol/l).
ii. What is the dog's estimated MAP?
iii. What test would be done next for a definitive diagnosis?
iv. What is the most likely disease causing the changes given above?
v. What is the mechanism of the likely etiology in this dog?

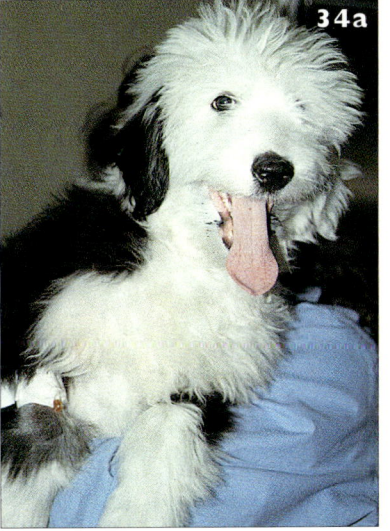

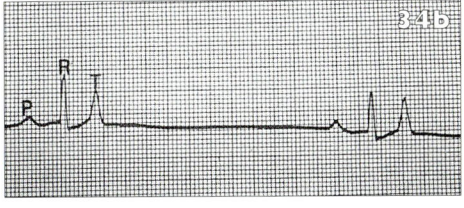

vi. What are the dangers of treating this crisis with corticosteroids prior to a definitive diagnosis?
vii. What is the initial treatment?
viii. Evaluate the ECG strip of this dog (**34b**).

33 & 34: Answers

33 i. The illuminated lateral equator of the displaced lens can be seen indicating the position of the lens in the anterior chamber.
ii. Secondary glaucoma due to anterior luxation of the lens.
iii. Because of the optic neuropraxia.
iv. Emergency therapy necessitates the reduction of the intraocular pressure to a physiological value. This can be achieved initially by using a hyperosmotic agent, providing the blood aqueous barrier is intact, but cure requires the emergency removal of the lens. The condition is inherited recessively and, although bilateral, there may be considerable delay between the first and second eye involvements.

34 i. b.
ii. Systolic pressure + (2 × diastolic pressure ÷ 3) = 68 mmHg (9.0kPa).
iii. ACTH stimulation test.
iv. Hypoadrenocorticism (Addison's disease).
v. Immunologic destruction of the adrenals is typically the cause, although the incident of warfarin toxicity would indicate a possible bleed destroying the glandular architecture.
vi. As long as dexamethasone is used there is no problem. If prednisolone is used prior to the ACTH stimulation test, this drug will interfere with the ACTH stimulation diagnosis.
vii. Large volumes of saline are needed for resuscitation. Corticosteroids are given for their mineralocorticoid effect.
viii. The ECG (**34b**) shows tall spiked T waves and prolonged P-R intervals with bradycardia. This is compatible with hyperkalemia in the dog.

35–37: Questions

35 This eight-year-old, intact male Chihuahua has a stiff, stilted gait, caudal abdominal pain and a bloody discharge dripping from the penis (35). He has a fever of 105°F (40.6°C) and has not eaten for 2 days. He tries to bite during rectal palpation.
i. What is your presumptive diagnosis?
ii. How can the diagnosis be confirmed?
iii. What are your treatment recommendations?

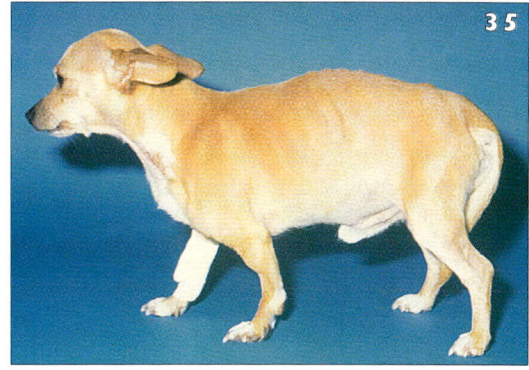

36 A one-year-old, male Fox Terrier is presented after having been kicked by a horse. The dog is tachypneic, and there is a section of thoracic wall on the left side which appears to move independently from the rest of the rib cage (36).
i. What is the likely diagnosis?
ii. What is your initial therapeutic plan?
iii. If your initial intervention does not improve the tachypnea and respiratory distress, what definitive therapy could you attempt?

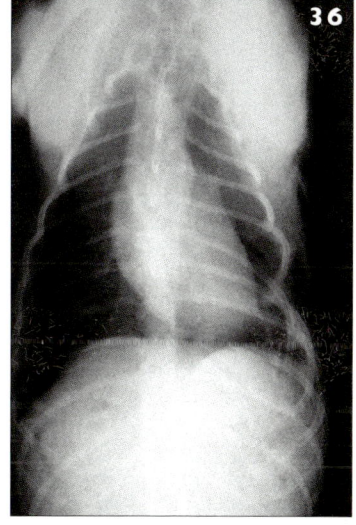

37 A ten-month-old, female Boxer is presented with a 1-day history of anxiety, running into walls and one episode of seizures. Previous history includes small bowel diarrhea of 3 days' duration 3 months ago and an episode of 'pneumonia' 1 month ago. The dog lives indoors and always walks outside on a leash. Physical examination is essentially normal. Neurologic examination reveals mental depression, disorientation, blindness and deafness.
i. What is your initial emergency management?
ii. What is the differential diagnosis?
iii. What is the diagnostic plan?
iv. How would you monitor and treat the condition?

35–37: Answers

35 i. Acute bacterial prostatitis.
ii. Physical examination reveals an enlarged, painful prostate gland. Hematology shows a neutrophilic leukocytosis with a left shift. Urinalysis usually shows RBCs, WBCs and bacteria in the urine. The diagnosis can be confirmed by culture and cytology of prostatic fluid, but ejaculation or prostatic wash may not be possible in dogs with extreme pain. Culture of the urine by cystocentesis is usually adequate to identify the organism. Radiography and ultrasonography are helpful in diagnosing prostatic abscesses.
iii. Treatment involves antibiotic therapy and supportive care with i/v fluids. Recommended antibiotics include erythromycin, clindamycin, trimethoprim-sulfa, chloramphenicol and the quinolones. Antibiotics should be continued for at least 21 days, or for 6–8 weeks for prostatic abscesses. Cessation of antibiotic therapy should be followed by negative culture. Castration is recommended to reduce prostatic tissue mass. Surgical drainage, in addition to antibiotic therapy and castration, is recommended for prostatic abscesses. Septic shock may occur if a prostatic abscess ruptures, requiring exploratory laparotomy, abdominal lavage and open peritoneal drainage as treatment for acute fulminant peritonitis.

36 i. The moving section of thoracic wall suggests a flail segment. This is caused by two or more fractures in two or more adjacent ribs causing a section of thoracic wall to be detached from the rib cage. The movement of the flail segment is typically described as paradoxical.
ii. Oxygen supplementation, analgesics and hemodynamic stabilization. If the dog is in severe respiratory distress, positive pressure ventilation is indicated. Thoracic radiographs should be taken to determine whether other concurrent intrathoracic injuries exist, e.g. pulmonary contusions, pneumothorax, hemothorax.
iii. The flail segment can be stabilized by securing it to the neighboring regions of the thoracic wall. Under local anesthesia, sutures can be placed around the flail segment ribs and anchored onto a splint constructed of tongue depressors, aluminum rods, orthoplast or other rigid materials. If general anesthesia is used, the patient should be maintained on gas anesthesia to allow mechanical ventilation during the procedure.

37 i. An i/v catheter is placed and anticonvulsant drugs such as diazepam are drawn and made ready to administer should seizure activity recur. An emergency data base is obtained to include glucose, PCV, TS, BUN, sodium and potassium.
ii. Should include: infectious diseases such as distemper; rabies; bacteria, fungal and rickettsial diseases; toxoplasmosis; and *Neosporum caninum* infection. Also, congenital abnormalities such as hydrocephalus or hepatoportal shunts; cardiovascular disease; toxic ingestion (such as lead, metaldehyde, ethylene glycol); metabolic diseases such as renal failure, liver failure, severe electrolyte abnormalities, glucose abnormalities; head trauma and brain tumor are possible.
iii. Complete neurologic and ophthalmologic examination should be performed. CBC, chemistry profile, urinalysis, blood ammonia, osmolar gap and blood lead levels may rule out some metabolic and toxic conditions. ECG monitoring can help assess cardiac disturbance. Serologic testing and CSF evaluation can help diagnose infectious diseases such as toxoplasmosis, distemper, rickettsial diseases, fungal diseases and *Neosporum caninum* infection. Organic brain disease may be detected by MRI or CT scan.
iv. Pending diagnostic information, the dog is treated symptomatically. I/v fluids, glucocorticoids at an anti-inflammatory dose and antibiotics that cross the blood–brain barrier (e.g. trimethoprim-sulfa and chloramphenicol) are given. Anticonvulsants are administered should seizure activity recur or persist.

38 & 39: Questions

38 A two-year-old, male German Shepherd Dog is presented for weakness, anorexia, weight loss and epistaxis. Physical examination findings: HR – 178 bpm; bounding femoral pulses; pale mucous membranes; CRT – 2 seconds; splenomegaly; unilateral epistaxis; and mild dehydration. The hemogram shows: WBCs – 3500/mm^3; PCV – 21%; platelets – 65,000/mm^3. 38 shows a peripheral blood smear.

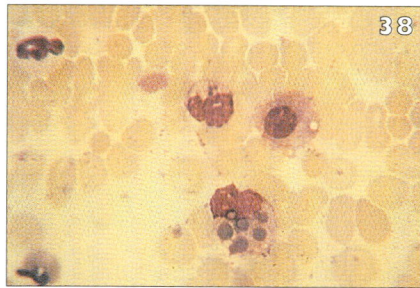

i. What are your immediate concerns?
ii. What is the differential diagnosis?
iii. What is the initial diagnostic and treatment plan?
iv. How would you treat the disease and prevent recurrence?
v. What is the long-term prognosis?

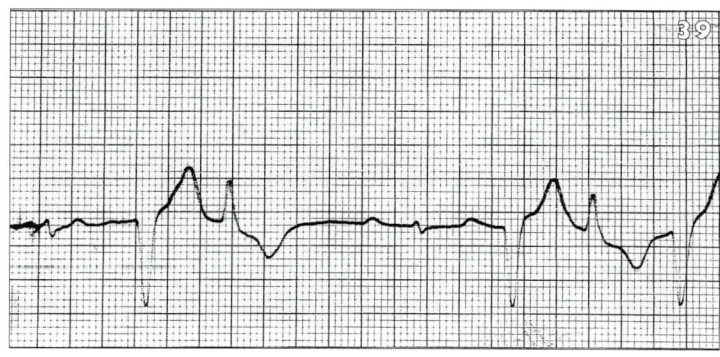

39 A mature, stray male cat is presented anorexic, dehydrated and febrile. An i/v catheter is placed and intravenous lactated Ringer's solution (LRS) is begun with an initial 150 ml bolus. In addition, i/v ampicillin is administered and the cat is placed in isolation. The following day the cat is markedly weak, depressed and has rapid shallow respiration; 700 ml of the LRS has been given. HR is rapid and pulse deficits are appreciated in addition to a grade IV murmur equally audible on the left and right. The lungs have mild crackles diffusely. Based on your assessment and the lead II ECG recorded at 50mm/sec (39):
i. What is your ECG diagnosis?
ii. What would be your approach to initial therapy?
iii. What are the possible causes of the murmur and apparent congestive failure?

38 & 39: Answers

38 i. Further blood loss due to thrombocytopenia, together with the concurrent anemia, will decrease oxygen delivery to tissues. Leukopenia is a risk factor for sepsis.
ii. Epistaxis could be a result of intranasal disease, trauma, infection, foreign body, neoplasia or extranasal causes, e.g. coagulopathy, increase in capillary permeability, hypertension. In this case the pancytopenia and splenomegaly increase the likelihood of canine ehrlichiosis (tropical pancytopenia), which is common in German Shepherd dogs, and may rule out other disease conditions. Other causes of pancytopenia are estrogen toxicity and myelophthisis.
iii. Hemostasis should be attempted by using cold packs or instilling dilute epinephrine (1:10,000) intranasally. Restricting the animal's activity and possibly administering a phenothiazine tranquilizer, which is a vasodilator and reduces BP, and administration of platelet rich plasma or fresh whole blood will arrest the bleeding. I/v fluids may be used to correct dehydration. Oxygen therapy should be given to improve tissue oxygenation. Broad-spectrum antibiotics may prevent the animal from becoming septic in the face of severe leukopenia.
iv. Long-term therapy includes two repetitive injections of imidocarb 10–14 days apart and oral oxytetracycline or doxycycline for 14–21 days. In case of bone marrow suppression due to prolonged exposure, corticosteroids are indicated. Careful tick control and prophylactic use of tetracyclines will help to prevent recurrence.
v. The prognosis depends on the chronicity and severity of the disease. Non-regenerative anemia and/or severe leukopenia are poor prognostic signs. The chronic stage of the disease and prolonged exposure to the parasite result in bone marrow hypoplasia or aplasia.

39 i. Ventricular rate approximately 140 bpm, with ventricular ectopic beats.
ii. Discontinue the i/v fluids and give an initial bolus of furosemide (2 mg/kg). Administer oxygen and immediately determine K^+, Ca^{++}, acid–base status, magnesium level. An echocardiogram would help evaluate cardiac muscle and chamber size and function.
iii. Fluid overload may explain the apparent pulmonary edema, though it is possible that there is also underlying heart disease. If a murmur was indeed present prior to fluid therapy, either HCM or possibly DCM exists, or bacterial endocarditis, though this is not commonly seen in cats. If bacterial endocarditis is suspected, it is likely the cat is FIV positive.

40 & 41: Questions

40 A six-year-old Somali cat was presented with a history of polyuria, polydipsia, weight loss, vomiting and lethargy (**40**). The cat had not been eating well for the past 3 days. Physical examination found the cat approximately 8% dehydrated and mentally depressed. There was evidence of weight loss. Thoracic and abdominal examination was unremarkable. The retinas were normal. Initial laboratory data: PCV – 55%; TS – 8.5 g/dl; BUN labstick – 50–80 mg/dl; glucose by labstick – 460 mg/dl (25,8 mmol/l); Na^+ – 165 mEq/l; K^+ – 2.6 mEq/l; venous pH – 7.2; PCO_2 – 40 mmHg; HCO_3 – 8 mEq/l. Urinanalysis: SG – 1.026

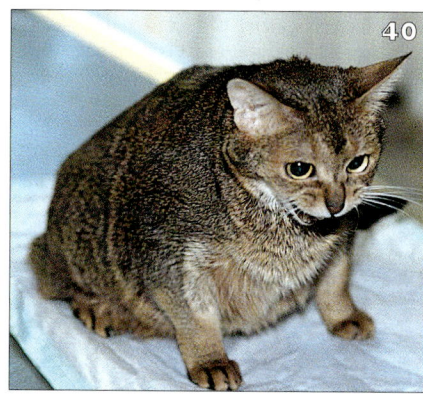

with 4+ glucose, 2+ ketones, 1+ protein, 5 WBCs/hpf and intracellular cocci. Initial BP by indirect methods was 120/80 mmHg (16/10.6 kPa).
i. What is your working diagnosis and problems list?
ii. Describe your initial treatment plan for this cat.
iii. What other electrolytes must you evaluate, and why?
iv. What are potential complications?
v. Would you use sodium bicarbonate? Why or why not?
vi. You are treating the cat and have brought the glucose to within normal range. However, there is now 4+ ketonuria. Explain the increase in ketones on the urine dipstick.

41 A nine-month-old Maltese Terrier is presented for having a seizure once at home 45 minutes ago. The dog is now alert and responsive (**41**). Vital signs are within normal limits. There is no previous history of seizures, though the owners confirm a history of previous episodes of behavioral abnormalities including circling, apparent blindness and ataxia over the last month.
i. Without referring to the clinical pathology results below, list the possible etiologies for this type of neurologic derangement in a young dog.
 Blood work shows microcytosis of red cells without anemia and low albumin, urea and cholesterol levels, and with normal liver enzymes. Ammonium biurate crystals are found in the urine.
ii. What is the likely diagnosis?
iii. What definitive diagnostics are appropriate for the differentials you listed in ii.?
iv. What specific hematological test should be performed before performing a liver biopsy in this patient?

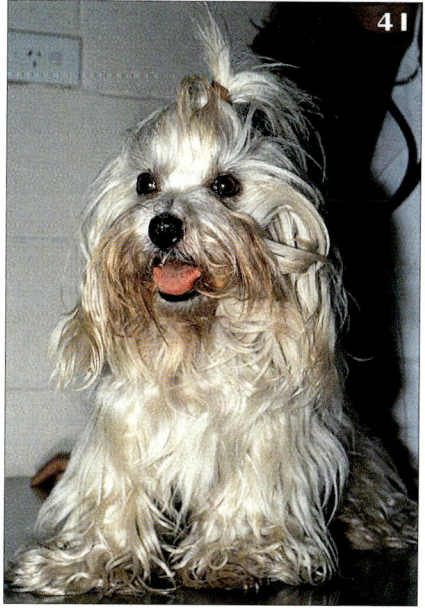

40 & 41: Answers

40 i. Diabetes mellitus with ketoacidosis. Problems include history of polyuria/polydipsia, anorexia and weight loss, azotemia, cystitis, dehydration, ketonuria, hyperglycemia.
ii. Rehydrate over 4–6 hours using a balanced electrolyte solution such as lactated Ringer's supplemented with potassium (5 mEq KCl/250 ml fluid) then maintenance fluids; after replacement of dehydration, initiate insulin therapy (regular insulin at 1 unit/kg/day); monitor blood glucose every 2 hours initially then every 4 hours; adjust insulin dosage, supplementing with glucose as needed, until glucose is in the range 150–200 mg/dl (8.4–11.2 mmol/l); i/v fluids are then changed to 2.5% dextrose in half-strength lactated Ringer's and the insulin is stopped; culture urine and begin bactericidal antibiotic effective against Gram-positive cocci that get high urine concentration (e.g. amoxicillin, ampicillin). Begin s/c insulin (NPH, Lente, or PZ1) once glucose rises again and cat is eating.
iii. Serum phosphorus, magnesium and potassium are critical electrolytes. Hypophosphatemia is often evident on day 2 or 3 of hospitalization and can be associated with intravascular hemolysis and weakness. Hypokalemia should be anticipated once insulin therapy is initiated, and potassium must be supplemented.
iv. Complications include severe acidosis, arrhythmias, altered mentation, acute renal failure, hypernatremia, dehydration, hypophosphatemia, hypoglycemia from therapy, hypokalemia, thromboemboli and infections.
v. Rehydration and reperfusion should be the initial mainstay of the acid–base therapy. Overzealous bicarbonate therapy can lead to alkaline overshoot, hypokalemia, hypocalcemia, paradoxical CSF acidosis, hypernatremia and hyperosmolality, and shift of the oxyhemoglobin dissociation curve.
vi. As the glucose is lowered, the ketones become metabolized. Beta-hydroxybutyric acid is not detected on the urine dipstick. There could have been a high concentration of this metabolite initially. It is then metabolized to acetoacetic acid and acetic acid, which are detected by the urine test strip. Therefore, it appears as though there is an increase in ketones.

41 i. D – dysplastic, degenerative (unlikely in this age of dog); A – anatomical/vascular: portosystemic shunt, hydrocephalus, vascular accident, anticoagulant ingestion and bleeding. M – metabolic: hypoglycemia, uremia; N – nutritional (hypocalcemia, thiamine deficient), neoplastic; I – infectious (parasitic, bacterial, protozoal, fungal), inflammatory (granulomatous meningoencephalitis, steroid-responsive meningoencephalitis), immune-mediated, iatrogenic, idiopathic; T – trauma, toxins (lead, ethylene glycol).
 The **DAMNIT** mnemonic is an effective way of categorizing etiologies and recalling specific differential diagnosis which may be applicable to a given systemic derangement. There is a microcytosis present in the red cell line, but no anemia. Low albumin, urea and cholesterol levels in the face of normal hepatic enzymes suggest decreased liver function without evidence of an inflammatory response or hepatocellular injury. Ammonium biurate crystals are formed in the urine as a result of high serum ammonia concentrations, which further supports the premise of a dysfunctional liver.
ii. These clinical pathology results support a diagnosis of hepatic encephalopathy, very likely due to a portosystemic shunt.
iii. An ultrasound study of the liver and associated vascular structures and liver biopsy. Exploratory laparotomy and a portovenogram would be necessary for definitive assessment of whether the shunt was extrahepatic or intrahepatic, and therefore repairable or not. Portal pressures are monitored during ligation procedures to guide the degree of ligation that will be tolerated by the patient.
iv. A clotting profile should be performed since the liver is largely responsible for the manufacture of clotting factors, and there may well be a deficiency of them if the liver is dysfunctional.

42 & 43: Questions

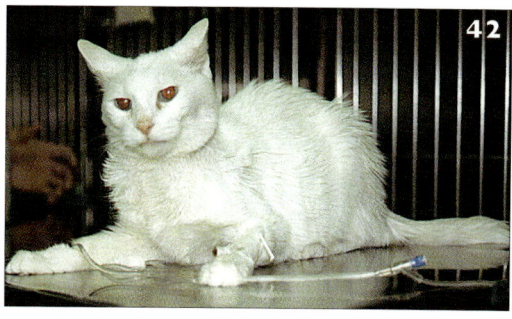

42 A nine-year-old, spayed female domestic cat is presented for an acute episode of open mouth breathing (42). The owner notes a history of polyuria and polydypsia in the past few weeks. There has been mild weight loss but no change in attitude or appetite until this evening. Primary survey reveals a relatively thin cat who is open mouth breathing and is very excited and restless. RR – 72 bpm; HR – 325 bpm; temperature –104.9°F (40.5°C); mucous membranes – pink; CRT – 0.5 second. A grade II/VI systolic murmur and an arrhythmia were auscultated. Lung sounds were normal in all lung fields. Dehydration was estimated at 5–8%.
An ECG revealed a sinus tachycardia with occasional atrial premature beats. Laboratory work incuded: PCV – 40%; TS – 6.5 g/dl; Na^+ – 148 mEq/l; K^+ – 4.4 mEq/l; chloride – 116 mEq/l; Ca^{++} (ionized) – 3.5 mEq/l; venous blood gas, pH – 7.30; $PvCO_2$ – 36 mmHg (4.8 kPa); PvO_2 – 56 mmHg (7.5 kPa); HCO_3 – 18 mEq/l; glucose – 180 mg/dl (10.1 mmol/l); creatinine – 2.2 mg/dl (194.5 µmol/l); T4 – 25 ng/ml (normal 1.2–4.8). Urinalysis: SG – 1.015, negative for glucose and ketones.
i. Which of the following is the most likely diagnosis for this cat?
a. Toxin ingestion. b. Thyroid storm. c. Septic shock. d. Congestive heart failure.
ii. What is the most appropriate therapy for the tachyarrhythmia?
a. Dobutamine. b. Propanolol. c. Enalapril. d. Furosemide.
iii. What mechanism does not contribute to the polyuria/polydypsia in this case?
a. Medullary washout. b. Increased glomerular filtration rate. c. Compulsive polydypsia. d. Osmotic diuresis.
iv. Which of the following statements is true? (select one)
a. A thyroid storm typically occurs when a hyperthyroid cat undergoes stress, such as a car ride. b. A hyperexcitable, hyperdynamic state is pathognomonic for ethylene glycol toxicity. c. The fever and tachycardia are a result of poor cardiac output associated with congestive heart failure. d. All of the above are true.

43 A ten-year-old domestic shorthair cat was taken to surgery for an exploratory laparotomy. A gastrostomy tube was placed at the time of surgery.
i. How soon can you start feeding? How would this time frame change if you had a jejunostomy tube in place? How can you tell if the amount being fed is being tolerated?
ii. What type of diet is best fed initially, and why?
iii. The cat had been anorectic for one week. When refeeding after a period of anorexia, how quickly should you achieve full caloric intake?
iv. What are the options for reaching the goal of full caloric intake with a liquid diet or with a canned diet?
v. What is the primary metabolic complication associated with refeeding an anorectic patient, and why does this occur?
vi. What is the difference between a polymeric and a monomeric diet? Why would you choose one over the other?
vii. How is caloric requirement estimated?

42 & 43: Answers

42 i. b.
ii. b.
iii. d.
iv. a.

43 i. Once the patient is alert enough so that regurgitation and silent aspiration will not occur. In addition, gastric motility may not be normal for 24–72 hours postoperatively and feeding may need to be withheld or proceed very slowly until that time. Jejunostomy tube feeding can be started immediately postoperatively.
ii. Liquid diets are recommended initially. Gastric motility may be impaired postoperatively, secondary to normal inhibition following a laparotomy or to the underlying disease. The stomach will be more likely to empty liquid than solids or gruels. Additionally, the tube can be aspirated intermittently and residuals measured.
iii. A minimum of 3 days.
iv. When an isosmotic liquid diet is being used the diet can be started at full strength and one third of the projected volume, and increased in increments of 30%/day. With hyperosmotic diets (liquids or solids) feedings should be diluted to attain an isosmotic concentration initially.
v. Hypophosphatemia. In response to feeding, phosphorus moves intracellularly because it is required for the synthesis of phosphorylated compounds. Insulin also promotes the uptake of phosphorus.
vi. Polymeric diets are made of complex carbohydrates and proteins and require digestion prior to absorption. Monomeric diets are elemental diets based on amino acids that require no digestion prior to absorption.
vii. Various formulas exist for calculating the resting energy requirement (RER). These are all approximations and should be used as guidelines only. (For instance, the patient suffering from chronic malnutrition may actually have a lower metabolic rate than anticipated.) A simple formula is $2(30 \times \text{body weight (kg)} + 70)$. It has been suggested this caloric value should be multiplied by a 'stress factor' based on the underlying disease. RER should be multiplied by 1.2 for minor surgery, trauma or illness; 1.5 for sepsis or major trauma; burn patients may require up to twice the RER.

44 & 45: Questions

44 A middle-aged, male dog presents for protracted vomiting of 2 days' duration. Palpation of the abdomen reveals painful intestines. A barium study reveals accordion-pleated small intestines suggesting a linear foreign body obstruction (**44a**). Upon surgical exploration the duodenum and proximal jejunum are accordion pleated and diffusely red with a few areas of blackened serosa along the mesenteric border.
i. The mouth should be thoroughly examined when this patient is anesthetized. Why?
ii. What are the surgical recommendations for removal of a linear foreign body?
iii. If there is a concern about healing over a particular anastamosis, what surgical procedures may reinforce the healing site?
iv. How much bowel can be removed without encountering significant postoperative changes such as chronic diarrhea and malnutrition?
v. What are the indications for feeding tube placement (**44b**)?
vi. Where can feeding tubes be placed?

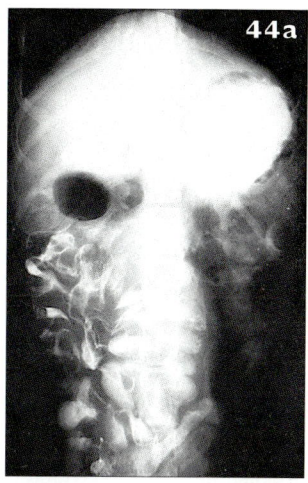

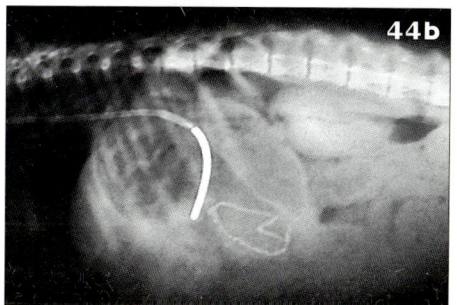

45 A patient presents with a limb amputation at the proximal tibia (**45**). The owners had been applying direct pressure to the wound. On removal of the towel there is evidence of a bleeding arterial vessel.
i. While you are getting ready to ligate the vessel, what temporary measure should be performed and with what?
ii. Name four methods of controlling bleeding to a wound on the distal hindlimb.
iii. A tourniquet should not be placed on the limb to control hemorrhage. Give three reasons why tourniquets should be avoided.
iv. True or false:
a. A severed artery will often stop bleeding spontaneously; therefore, if continuous bleeding is seen, the vessel must be partially torn.
b. If direct ligation of a bleeding artery does not control severe hemorrhage, the artery supplying the entire area should be ligated.
c. Persistent arterial hemorrhage can often be controlled with a compressive bandage.
d. Persistent venous hemorrhage can often be controlled with a compressive bandage.

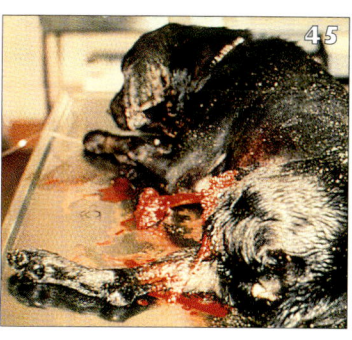

44 & 45: Answers

44 i. To inspect the tongue for attachment of the linear foreign body. If it is present, its attachment should be cut.

ii. The proximal end of the linear foreign body should be milked through the intestines and into the colon. If it is not able to be milked down, the proximal end should be removed via a gastrotomy or enterotomy over the site of attachment. There are several ways to remove the remaining end: either by performing multiple enterotomies over the antimesenteric side of the intestines and removing sections of the linear foreign body; or by tying the proximal end to a tube and milking the tube through the intestines into the colon where it should be digitally removed via the rectum before closure of the abdomen. The intestines that have blackened mesenteric serosa should be resected and anastamosed. Any suspected areas of infarction or devitalized tissue should also be removed, or have serosal patching performed over them.

iii. A serosal patch can be performed by opposing the serosa just outside the incision on either side of the incision with interrupted sutures, or by tacking serosa of other small bowel over the anastamosis with interrupted sutures. The omentum can also be tacked over the questionable anastamosis.

iv. 70–80%

v.
- Patient unable to take food via oral alimentation (facial fractures, dental procedures, vomiting, esophageal stricture).
- Known anorexia or malnutrition (metabolic problem, neoplasia) with no immediate resolution anticipated.
- Diseased/malfunctioning GI tract (large resection, neoplasia).
- Animal unwilling to eat.

vi. Orogastric (temporary); nasoesophageal, nasogastric, nasojejunal; pharyngostomy; esophagostomy; gastrostomy; gastrojejunal; duodenal; jejunal.

45 i. Direct pressure should be reapplied using sterile material.

ii. Direct pressure to the wound; pressure to the femoral artery by placing pressure in the inguinal and femoral canal region; use of a blood pressure cuff inflated proximal to the wound; direct ligation of blood vessels.

iii. Pressure on neurovascular bundles can lead potentially to permanent neurologic damage; ischemia, which may be irreversible, can occur to tissues distal to tourniquet; thromboses are possible.

iv. a – true; b – true; c – false; d – true.

46–48: Questions

46 This three-year-old male Boxer (**46**) had a history of acute abdominal pain and vomiting. He appeared anorexic and 6% dehydrated. Abdominal radiographs revealed enlarged kidneys. The CBC and biochemical profile showed normal values. The urinalysis found: SG – 1.035; protein – 2+; blood – 1+; sediment – >10 WBCs per high power field and WBC casts.
i. What is your tentative diagnosis?
ii. What other diagnostic tests are indicated?
iii. Outline the therapeutic goals for this patient.
iv. What should be done if the pyuria persists?

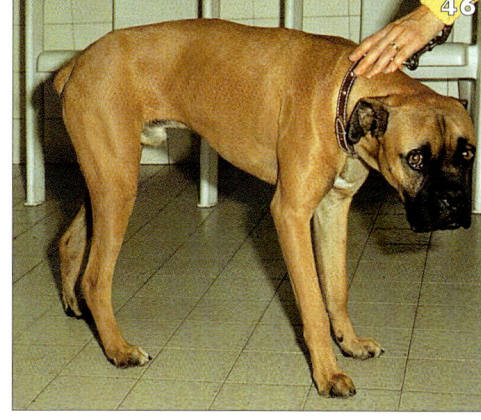

47 A 'ready' area that allows the staff immediate access to materials necessary for immediate life-saving resuscitation is shown (**47**).
i. What materials should be ready for cardiopulmonary resuscitation?
ii. What materials should be ready for resuscitation of severe respiratory failure?

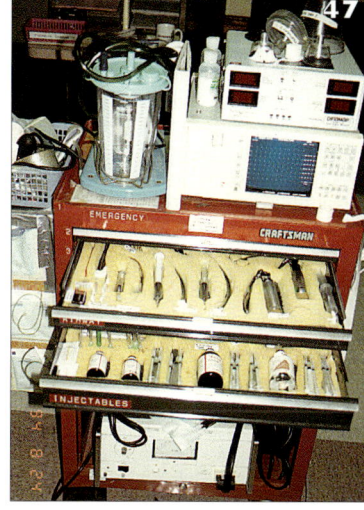

48 A middle-aged, male cat presents to the emergency clinic after falling from a fifth-storey window. The cat is in the middle stage of shock with no obvious fractures. After initial fluid resuscitation the intensive care unit nurse alerts you that the cat has urinated a moderate amount of bloody urine.
i. What are the clinical and laboratory signs of renal trauma?
ii. What radiographic signs are suggestive of renal trauma on plain and contrast radiographs?
iii. During surgical exploration, evidence of a perirenal hematoma is discovered. What are the indications for exploration of the hematoma?
iv. After exploration and repair of an expanding subcapsular renal hematoma, what procedure will prevent postoperative twisting of the kidney?

46–48: Answers

46 i. The abdominal pain, urine sediment and enlarged kidneys are compatible with acute pyelonephritis. However, acute nephrotoxicity such as ethylene glycol should be a differential diagnosis and ruled in or out.
ii. Careful history for exposure to potential renal toxins, ethylene glycol test and osmolar gap if exposure or history is compatible; intravenous excretory urogram; urinary tract ultrasound; urinary culture by cystocentesis; search for underlying focus of infection and any evidence of urinary tract calculi or diverticuli.
iii. Therapy is based on long-term antibiotic therapy as indicated by bacterial culture and sensitivity. Antibiotics are given for a minimum of 4 weeks. Supportive therapy consists of: fluid therapy, control of urinary pH and monitoring for renal impairment or failure.
iv. The urine should be monitored for infection, with urine cultures during therapy. Changes in antibiotic selection may be required. Low-dose, long-term antibiotic therapy (>6 months) may be necessary.

47 i.
- *Airway* – endotracheal tubes (variety of sizes) loaded with air-filled syringes; gauze to tie in tubes; tracheostomy tubes; laryngoscope with three sizes of blades; suction unit; several sizes and lengths of suction tips; scalpel blades.
- *Breathing* – AMBU bag; oxygen source with oxygen tubing.
- *Circulation* – catheters for i/v or i/o access; tape; caps; clippers; electrical defibrillator; ECG; BP monitoring device; syringes (1 ml, 3 ml, 12 ml) preloaded with needles; drugs (epinephrine, calcium gluconate, atropine, bretylium, methylprednisolone, lidocaine, dopamine, dobutamine, crystalloids, 250 ml bags 5% dextrose in water); surgical pack with rib spreaders. Additional monitoring equipment might include a pulse oximeter and an end-tidal CO_2 monitor.

ii. Same as **i.** above for airway, breathing and circulation plus doyen forceps for retrieval of foreign bodies; mouth gags in several sizes; 19G butterfly catheter, 3-way stopcock and 60 ml syringe connected for rapid thoracocentesis; chest tubes of several sizes; underwater chest drainage suction system (Heimlich valve for large dogs only if no suction available); small surgical pack; drugs for sedation such as narcotics and tranquilizers.

48 i.
- Microscopic or gross hematuria.
- Elevated BUN, creatinine, potassium.
- Oliguria, anuria.
- Non-responsive shock.
- Painful paralumbar region.

ii. Loss of detail in the retroperitoneal space on plain radiographs.
Lack of contrast blush of the kidneys during excretory urogram.
Loss of contrast into the retroperitoneal space on excretory urogram.
Normal plain radiographs.
iii. Pulsation of the hematoma and evidence of hematoma expansion.
iv. Tacking the capsule or kidney with non-absorbable suture to the body wall in a position that places the least amount of stress on the blood supply and prevents kinking and obstruction of the vessels and ureter.

49 & 50: Questions

49 A three-year-old, entire male German Shepherd Dog is recovering from surgery for gastric dilatation/volvulus performed last night. He has vomited several times, including once immediately following extubation, and seems to be depressed. RR – 76 bpm; HR – 140 bpm with a regular rhythm; temperature – 103.5°F (39.7°C). Crackles are auscultated over the right ventral thorax.
i. What is the radiographic diagnosis (**49**)?
ii. What is the most likely etiology of this condition?
iii. What medical therapies will you initiate, and how do you make this decision?
iv. What additional nursing practices could be included which may aid in treating this specific diagnosis?

50 A 12-year-old, spayed female Himalayan cat is presented because of vomiting and anorexia (**50a**). The owner reports that the cat has been inappetent and losing weight for approximately 2 weeks; the cat now weighs 5.8 kg. Physical examination reveals pale, icteric mucous membranes; CRT – 2 seconds; temperature – 101.3°F (38.5°C); HR – 180 bpm; RR – 24 bpm. The cat appears to be moderately overweight, in spite of the owner's insistence on recent weight loss. You estimate that the cat is 5% dehydrated. Abdominal palpation reveals a large, firm, non-painful liver. You decide to run a full hemogram, serum chemistry profile and urinalysis. There is a mature leukocytosis and an elevation in serum alkaline phosphatase and bilirubin. There is bilirubinuria. PCV = 22%; TS = 8.5 g/dl.

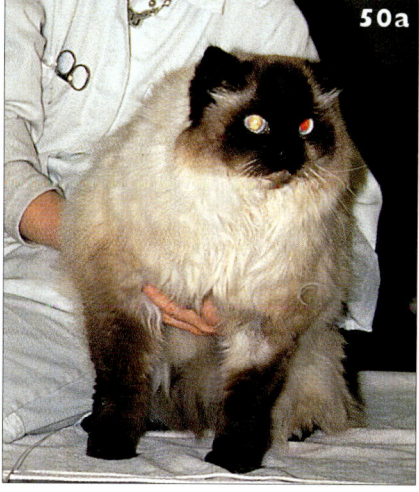

i. Give the cat's initial problems list, and interpret the clinical pathology results. What are the differential diagnoses? How would you differentiate the choices?
ii. What are the key considerations in fluid therapy of this patient and disease?
iii. Are systemic antibiotics appropriate in the management of this patient?
iv. Nutritional support and management are crucial in the management of this patient's disease. List and describe two methods of tube feeding that might be used, and list some considerations for the diet to be provided.

49 & 50: Answers

49 i. The most likely diagnosis is pneumonia.
ii. The cranioventral distribution and the history of vomiting are supportive of aspiration pneumonia.
iii. Antibiotic therapy should be initiated based on initial Gram stain of a transtracheal aspirate sample. The sample should be submitted for aerobic culture and antibiotic sensitivity testing. If the animal is too distressed to tolerate a transtracheal aspirate, an i/v broad-spectrum bactericidal antibiotic combination (e.g. ampicillin and gentamicin) would be appropriate.
iv. Nebulization with sterile saline (± antibiotics), coupage of the thoracic walls and strict attention to overall hydration status are important to keep the airways moist and encourage clearance of debris. Nutritional support should be implemented.

50 i. Vomiting, anorexia, dehydration, weight loss. The clinical pathology indicates a working diagnosis of cholestatic liver disease with mild dehydration and a secondary anemia. Changes in the leukogram are attributable to stress. Differential diagnoses include extrahepatic bile duct occlusion, hepatic lipidosis, cholangiohepatitis, hepatic neoplasia.

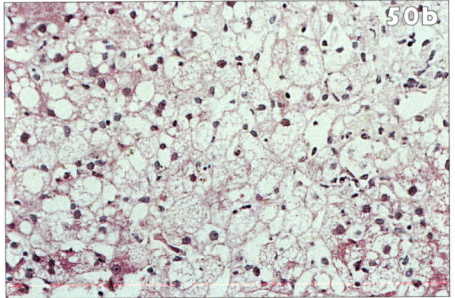

Differentiation of the choices could be accomplished provisionally by abdominal ultrasound and confirmed by percutaneous liver biopsy. In liver disease of this magnitude, it would be critical to assess a clotting profile and/or give prophylactic vitamin K1 prior to biopsy. This patient has hepatic lipidosis (**50b**)
ii. The cat should be rehydrated with a balanced electrolyte solution such as Plasma-Lyte. It is not advisable to supplement glucose in the i/v fluids since this can lead to increased fat storage within the liver cells. Potassium levels should be monitored twice daily, and hypokalemia corrected. Inorganic phosphorus levels must be monitored for hypophosphatemia which can lead to acute hemolysis. Potassium phosphate therapy would be indicated. Water soluble and fat soluble (A, D, E and K) vitamins are recommended for any cat with lipidosis. Particular attention is given to thiamine supplementation (50–100 mg/cat/day).
iii. Antibiotics (amoxicillin and metronidazole) are indicated in patients with hepatic insufficiency. The dose of metronidazole is conventionally reduced by half in severe liver disease. Tetracyclines, chloramphenicol and trimethoprim-sulfas should be avoided.
iv. Either an esophagostomy or gastrostomy tube would be appropriate for this patient. Force feeding by mouth is not likely to be an effective solution. Nasogastric tube feeding restricts the kind of diet that can be fed due to the necessary small diameter in the cat. The aim of nutritional support for a cat with hepatic lipidosis is to provide enough calories so that peripheral lipolysis and protein catabolism are inhibited, but not so many that lipid storage begins to occur. The calories should be sufficient to meet maintenance energy requirement (about 60–80 cal/kg/day).

The diet should contain only about 10% fat (dry weight basis) and 3–4 g protein/kg body weight. A high-quality commercial feline diet such as C/D® or Nutritional Recovery Formula® will provide the necessary balance of fat and protein and is preferred as long as signs of hepatic encephalopathy are not present. Supplementation with arginine, taurine and carnitine is recommended.

51 & 52: Questions

51 This seven-year-old Chihuahua (**51**) is currently being treated for pancreatitis with i/v lactated Ringer's solution, nasogastric suctioning and pain relief. The critical care nurse alerts you that the dog's HR has increased from 120 to 180 bpm and his CRT is now rapid (<1 sec). His pulses are bounding and his mucous membrane color is dark red. He recently received a butorphanol injection for pain.
i. What stage of shock is this animal in (compensatory, early decompensatory, decompensatory)? Justify your selection.
ii. What is the pathophysiologic mechanism responsible for these cardiovascular changes?

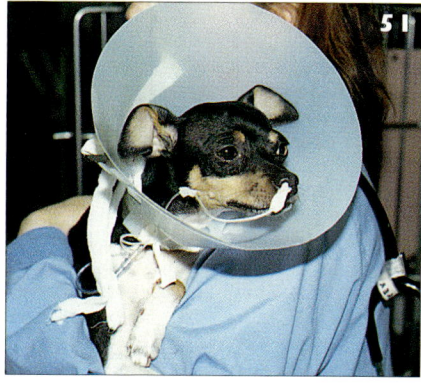

iii. The dog has a serum albumin of 1.4 g/dl (normal 3.0–4.0 g/dl). Give the pros and cons of the following fluids related to this laboratory value: hetastarch, dextran-40, plasma, dextran-70, gelatins.

52 This 12-year-old, male Rottweiler presented for gastric dilatation (**52**). The patient was resuscitated, surgery performed and a nasogastric feeding tube placed to initiate enteral feeding postoperatively.
i. Explain the benefits of nutritional support and enteral feeding to the SIRS or septic patient.
ii. What are the neuroendocrine and biochemical changes noted with the hypermetabolic state of sepsis or SIRS?
iii. What are the advantages of glutamine and arginine supplementation in diets for septic patients?

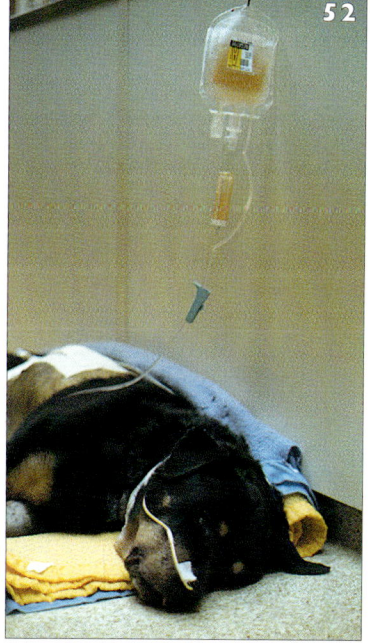

51 & 52: Answers

51 i. Compensatory, based on the increased HR, rapid CRT, dark red mucous membranes and bounding pulses.
ii. An acute loss of intravscular volume in this dog leads to decreased venous return, decreased cardiac output and decreased baroreceptor stretch. Increased sympathetic output occurs, causing an increase in SVR, vasoconstriction, HR and contractility. Venous return is increased by movement of interstitial water into the intravascular space, venoconstriction and renal water retention. Arterial blood flow is increased as cardiac output and SVR are increased.
iii. Albumin loss in this case may be a result of third spacing into the GI tract and peripheral tissues as a result of SIRS-related vasculitis. The holes in the endothelium have become large enough to allow loss of the 69,000 Dalton molecule albumin. A decrease in serum albumin causes a decrease in intravascular colloid oncotic pressure. The ideal replacement fluid for albumin levels below 2.0 g/dl is albumin (in the form of plasma), not only for oncotic support, but also for drug, electrolyte and hormonal carrying capacity. However, because the vessels are still leaky, additional oncotic support is necessary, preferably with a molecule larger than 69,000 Daltons such as hetastarch. Dextran-40 and gelatins are low molecular weight colloids and will leak through smaller holes than albumin, making them ineffective at maintaining intravascular oncotic pressure in the long term. Dextran-70 does not offer any benefit over albumin.

52 i. The SIRS patient is in a hypermetabolic state which will lead to protein catabolism, a negative energy balance state, decreased skeletal, cardiac and organ muscle strength, compromised immune defenses and potential bacterial translocation. Early nutritional support will alleviate these complications. Enteral nutritional support is important in order to adequately nourish the enterocytes. Without adequate enteral nutrition, the enterocytes will die and slough, leading to a higher risk of bacterial translocation.
ii. Neuroendocrine changes involve activation of the sympathetic nervous system, stimulation of the hypothalamic-pituitary-adrenal axis and an increase in glucagon secretion relative to insulin. Biochemical changes are secondary to inflammatory mediators and cytokines.
iii. Glutamine – very important energy source for the enterocytes, lymphocytes and fibroblasts. Thus glutamine aids in preventing bacterial translocation and in immune function and wound repair. Arginine – important for nitrogen retention and improved immune system function.

53 & 54: Questions

53 A two-year-old cat had come from the garden in blepharospasm (**53**). The owners could not open the eyelids and immediately sought your help because they considered the cat to be in pain. How would you pursue a diagnosis in this patient?

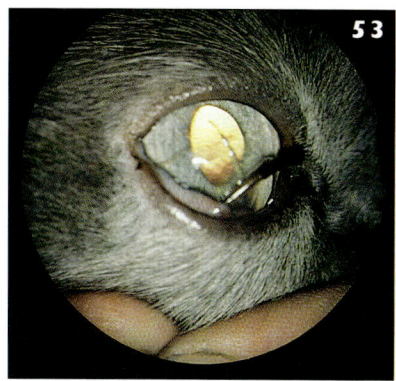

54 This four-year-old, spayed female dog presented with an acute onset of profuse hemorrhagic diarrhea (**54**). She had vomited once prior to the onset of diarrhea. Her vaccination history was up-to-date and there were no recent changes in diet or known exposure to garbage or toxins. She was depressed; mucous membranes were dry and pink with a rapid (<1 second) CRT. Skin turgor was normal. HR was 176 bpm with decreased

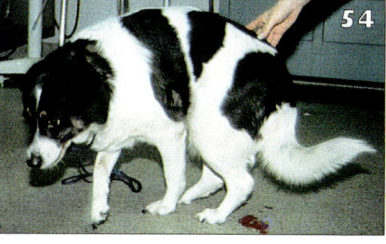

femoral pulse quality. Metatarsal pulses could not be palpated. The abdomen was 'doughy' on palpation. There was no localized pain nor palpable foreign body or mass. PCV – 69%; TS – 6.5 g/dl; BUN labstick = 30–40 mg/dl; glucose – 80 mg/dl (4.5 mmol/l).
i. What is your working diagnosis for the dog?
ii. In evaluating the fluid status in this patient, which of the following statements is most correct?
a. Fluid loss from the interstitial space leading to dehydration can be estimated accurately by skin turgor.
b. Fluid loss from the intravascular compartment is much greater than fluid loss from the interstitial compartment.
c. Fluid loss from the intravascular compartment is much less than fluid loss from the interstitial compartment.
d. Fluid loss from the intravascular compartment is approximately equal to that from the interstitial compartment.
iii. An i/v catheter was placed, and the dog given crystalloids and colloids at a rapid rate. What physical examination and monitoring parameters should be used to access restoration of adequate perfusion?
iv. An arterial blood gas sample was collected prior to initiation of therapy: pH – 7.12; PaO_2 – 85 mmHg (11.3 kPa); $PaCO_2$ – 34 mmHg (4.5 kPa); HCO_3 – 12.4 mEq/l. What is your interpretation of these findings?
v. Your calculations indicate that there is a high anion gap acidosis. What is the most likely source of unmeasured anion in this patient?
vi. Which of the following would be the best therapy to correct the acidosis in this patient: hyperventilation; sodium bicarbonate; rapid volume replacement; high flow O_2.
vii. Name three other causes of a high anion gap (normochloremic) acidosis.

53 & 54: Answers

53 Blepharospasm always complicates adequate clinical examination. In this instance it was overcome by using a combination of an auriculopalpebral nerve block and a topical anesthetic (proxymetacaine hydrochloride). Nothing abnormal could be seen initially and the cornea was fluorescein negative. Examination behind the membrana nictitans revealed a small piece of fishing line. Its removal effected immediate cure.

54 i. Hemorrhagic gastroenteritis.
ii. b.
iii. HR, CRT, peripheral pulse quality, BP, CVP, mentation.
iv. Partially compensated metabolic acidosis. The pH of 7.12 represents an acidemia. The low bicarbonate value indicates a metabolic acidosis. The low PCO_2 indicates a respiratory alkalosis. Because the dog is acidemic, the metabolic acidosis is assumed to be the primary disorder. The change in PCO_2 is within the expected range of compensation of the metabolic acidosis.
v. Lactate. Lactic acid accumulation secondary to decreased perfusion and anaerobic metabolism in the hypoxic tissues. However, exposure to toxins causing an increase in unmeasured anions cannot be ruled out.
vi. Rapid volume replacement.
vii. Ingestion of toxins such as ethylene glycol, ethanol, methanol; salicylate intoxication; diabetic ketoacidosis; uremic acidosis.

55 & 56: Questions

55 A five-year-old, castrated male domestic shorthair cat is presented after a 2 month history of slowly progressive dyspnea and anorexia. The owner is concerned today because the cat is coughing. On presentation the cat is tachypneic, with a RR of 60 bpm. Lung sounds are not auscultated in the ventral fields and the heart is muffled. The cat has a choppy, dysynchrous breathing pattern.
i. What is your initial emergency therapeutic plan?
ii. Thoracocentesis initially relieves the cat's distress and yields the fluid shown (55). What is the most likely character of this fluid, and how would you confirm this?
iii. What is your differential diagnosis for conditions associated with this type of fluid production?
iv. How would you proceed to determine the underlying disease process?
v. What are the therapeutic options and the prognosis for successful long-term management?

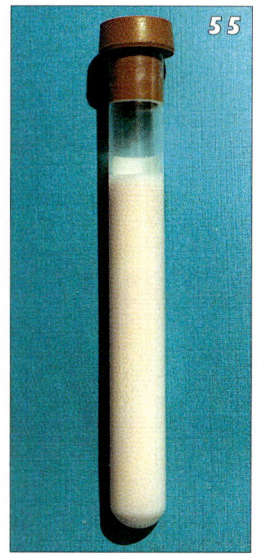

56 This three-year-old, castrated male Golden Retriever was shot during a walk in the woods (56). He had a large wound on the lateral side of his elbow and was brought to the emergency clinic immediately after the shooting. On presentation he was alert, had pink mucous membranes, had an open wound on the right elbow which was oozing dark blood, and was non-weightbearing lame on the left forelimb. Initial indirect BP measurements were 180/150 mmHg (24/20 kPa). He was started on i/v fluids, given oxymorphone to diminish the severe pain, and the wound was covered with a sterile bandage while radiographs were taken.
i. What initial diagnostics would you perform?
ii. What are probable causes for the mild hypertension?
iii. What is your radiographic interpretation of this limb?
iv. What is the treatment?

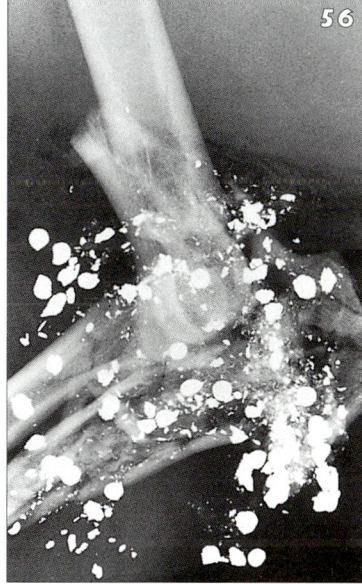

55 & 56: Answers

55 i. If the cat is dyspneic, oxygen supplementation is warranted. Thoracocentesis is indicated due to the muffled lung and heart sounds and breathing pattern.
ii. The appearance of the fluid is consistent with chylous effusion. The fluid should be analyzed for triglyceride and cholesterol content finding low cholesterol content when compared to serum. The cellular components are predominantly small lymphocytes and some neutrophils. Chyle does not settle upon centrifugation, but clears partially when mixed with ether.
iii. Chylothorax in cats has been associated with mediastinal lymphoma, heartworm disease, cardiomyopathy and trauma, although the majority are not found to have an obvious underlying cause and are termed idiopathic.
iv. The diagnostic approach to determine an underlying cause should include thoracic radiographs (following fluid evacuation by thoracocentesis or tube thoracostomy), CBC, serum biochemistry, heartworm test, FeLV and FIV tests, and echocardiography.
v. Treatment of the underlying disease process (e.g. improved cardiac function for cardiomyopathy, chemotherapy for lymphosarcoma) often leads to resolution of chylothorax. Medical management involves tube thoracostomy to allow continued drainage, and dietary management with a low fat diet and supplementation with short- or medium-chain fatty acids. Surgical options for therapy include thoracic duct ligation or the implantation of diaphragmatic mesh, pleuroperitoneal or pleurovenous shunts and pleurodesis. The prognosis is guarded as chylous effusion may not resolve and constrictive pleuritis may develop.

56 i. The skin must be examined for other penetrating wounds. It will be necessary to clip the dog's hair to undertake a thorough examination. Right forelimb, chest and survey abdominal films are important to detect penetrating trauma to a body cavity. A minimal data base of PCV, TS, BUN and glucose is necessary before attempting any kind of surgical intervention.
ii. Pain and compensatory shock.
iii. Gunshot wound to the elbow; severely comminuted articular fracture of the distal humerus, proximal radius and ulna.
iv. The comminution of this fracture is too extensive to try to reconstruct a functional articulation. There are two alternatives:
• Try to preserve the function of the limb with an arthrodesis. Preliminary treatment in this case is very extensive. Bullet trauma can cause severe tissue destruction, therefore the wounds should be thoroughly debrided; devitalized tissue and foreign bodies (bullets, hair and other debris) should be removed. The definitive orthopedic repair is delayed until infection is under control and non-viable tissue is eliminated. Prolonged hospital stay and multiple debridement procedures have to be expected. Failure of the final reconstruction is possible.
• Forelimb amputation. Debridement of the wound is still necessary, if amputation is delayed, to reduce the risk of sepsis.

57 & 58: Questions

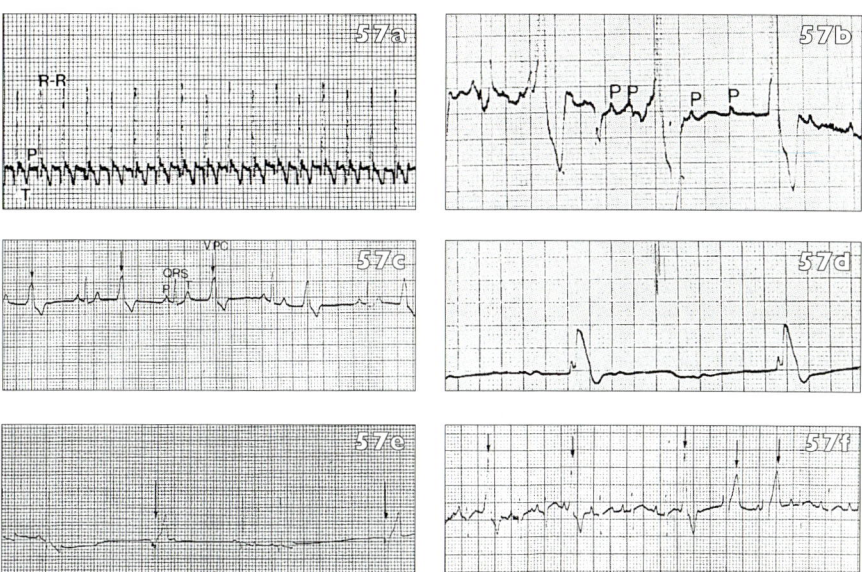

57 i. Match the arrhythmias (57a–57f) with the diagnoses listed at the right.
ii. How would you treat each arrhythmia?

Bigeminy
Third degree heart block
Atrial tachycardia
Sinus arrest with escape beats
Multiform ventricular ectopic beats
Idioventricular rhythm

58 The most common route of intoxication is ingestion.
i. For most toxins, induction of emesis is effective within what period of time after ingestion?
ii. Induction of emesis is commonly utilized in patients that have ingested a toxin. What are the contraindications to induction of emesis?
iii. A variety of emetics are employed in emergency veterinary medicine. Three commonly suggested emetics include Syrup of Ipecac, hydrogen peroxide and apomorphine. Comment on the dose, advantages and disadvantages of each of these emetics.
iv. Gastric lavage is also an effective way to decontaminate the stomach. What are the indications for gastric lavage?
v. After induction of emesis and/or gastric lavage, what other methods may be employed to prevent further absorption of ingested toxins?

57 & 58: Answers

57 i.

Bigeminy	c
3rd degree heart block	b
Atrial tachycardia	a
Sinus arrest with escape beats	e
Multiform ventricular ectopic beats	f
Idioventricular rhythm	d

ii. All need oxygen and treatment of underlying problem.
Bigeminy: oxygen, treat underlying problem, lidocaine if associated with poor perfusion.
3rd degree heart block: in emergency try atropine or isoproterenol; will need pacemaker.
Atrial tachycardia: carotid sinus massage; diltiazem if persistent.
Sinus arrest with escape beats: atropine or isoproterenol; may need pacemaker.
Multiform ventricular ectopic beats: lidocaine or procainamide.
Idioventricular rhythm: CPCR, dexamethasone.

58 i. Within 2–4 hours of ingestion for most toxins.
ii. Ingestion of a caustic material; patients with respiratory distress; patients that have a depressed gag reflex; patients that are likely to seizure; patients that are extremely weak, neurologically impaired or have laryngeal paralysis; bradycardic patients.
iii. Syrup of Ipecac (1.0–2.5 ml/kg p/o in the dog and 3.3 ml/kg p/o in the cat). Cats may find Syrup of Ipecac objectionable, and a 50:50 dilution with water may help alleviate this problem. The advantage of this drug is that it is readily available. Disadvantages include emesis possibly being delayed for as long as 20 minutes, and side-effects such as cardiotoxicity, hemorrhagic diarrhea and skeletal muscle weakness. The side-effects have been reported mainly with the use of the fluid extract or with chronic use. This formulation is no longer available.

Hydrogen peroxide induces emesis by local gastric irritation. The dose is 1–2 ml/kg (3% solution) p/o for the dog and cat. This dose may be repeated after 10 minutes if emesis has not occurred. The ability to produce emesis is inconsistent.

Apomorphine is the most reliable of the three. The dose of apomorphine in dogs is 0.03 mg/kg i/v or 0.04 mg/kg i/m. Topical application at 0.3 mg/kg is as effective as the same dose s/c. The advantage of the conjunctival route is ease of administration, and the effects of the apomorphine may be titrated to some extent by rinsing the conjunctival sac after vomiting has occurred. Mild conjunctivitis and sedation are common side-effects.
iv. When emesis is contraindicated or emetic induction was ineffective.
v. Oral administration of activated charcoal. A dose of 1–4 g/kg in 50–200 ml water is often recommended. Charcoal capsules may be used instead but are reported to be 25% less adsorptive than powders. A single dose of activated charcoal will suffice for many toxins. For toxins that undergo enterohepatic circulation, a dose every 4–6 hours combined with a cathartic may hasten elimination.

59–61: Questions

59 Epistaxis in this two-year-old Labrador-cross occurred 24 hours following suspected ingestion of warfarin (**59**).
i. Describe a diagnostic plan to confirm that this patient's epistaxis is warfarin-associated.
ii. How would you treat this patient?

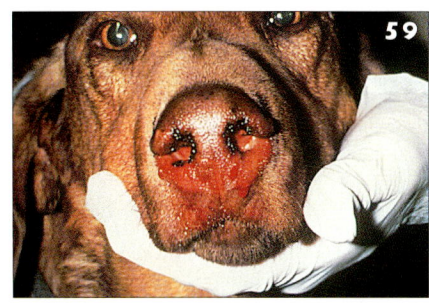

60 An 18-month-old Golden Retriever presents collapsed. HR – 80 bpm; femoral pulses weak and there is no dorsal pedal pulse (**60**). CRT – 2 seconds; mucous membranes are gray; 12% dehydrated; sodium – 130 mEq/l; chloride – 98 mEq/l; potassium – 8.2 mEq/l. The ECG shows tall spiked T waves, prolonged PR interval, widened QRS complex and a decrease in amplitude and widening of the P wave.
i. What fluid choice and what rate of administration would you use?

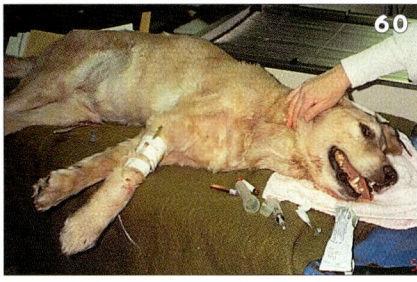

ii. What is an unusual finding in this patient that is 12% dehydrated?
iii. What is the likely diagnosis and what is the cause of the electrolyte disturbance?
iv. List possible causes of hyperkalemia.
v. Outline a treatment plan for life-threatening hyperkalemia.

61 This three-year-old bitch developed a purulent vaginal discharge 8 weeks after receiving estrogen therapy for pregnancy termination (**61**). For the past 2 days she has been febrile, lethargic, depressed, anorexic, polyuric and polydipsic. The following database was obtained: PCV – 48%; TS – 8.5 g/dl; BUN – 80 mg/dl; glucose – 100 mg/dl (5.6 mmol/l); Na – 148 mEq/l; K – 4.5 mEq/l; WBC – 40,000/ml^3. Urinalysis: SG – 1.023; sediment – 4+ RBCs, 4+ WBCs, rod bacteria; 3+ protein on dipstick.
i. What is your presumptive diagnosis?
ii. What factors predispose to this condition?
iii. What medical treatment options are available?
iv. What is your assessment of the bitch's renal function?

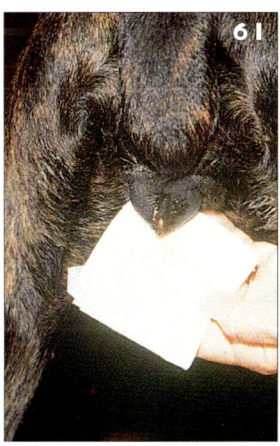

59–61: Answers

59 i. The diagnostic approach to the bleeding patient should include a platelet count, peripheral blood smear, PCV and ACT. Prolongation of the PT prior to prolongation of the PTT is consistent with warfarin ingestion. Because of the short half-life of factor VII, the PT, which evaluates the extrinsic coagulation system, is the most sensitive indicator of vitamin K-deficient coagulopathies. A positive assay for the presence of proteins induced by vitamin K antagonists (PIVKA) confirms the diagnosis.
ii. Treatment of animals with vitamin K-deficient coagulopathies varies with the severity of clinical signs. In animals with less severe signs, administration of supplemental vitamin K1 may be the only treatment necessary. Vitamin K1 should be administered i/m or s/c initially (5 mg/kg loading dose) followed by oral administration (2.5–5.0 mg/kg divided bid or tid). The duration of vitamin K supplementation is dependent on the generation of rodenticide consumed. With short-acting compounds such as warfarin, vitamin K supplementation is necessary for 7 days; long-acting compound ingestion (brodifacoum, diphacinone, bromadiolone) requires longer supplementation (up to 30 days). Severe hemorrhage will require fresh frozen plasma or fresh whole blood administration. When hemothorax impairs breathing, oxygen supplementation and thoracentesis can be life-saving.

60 i. Normal saline. If using crystalloids alone, 90 ml/kg/hour may be required.
ii. The low heart rate with poor pulse pressure.
iii. Hypoadrenocorticism (Na:K ratio of 16:1 – <27:1 is highly suspect). Hypoaldosteronism of Addison's diseases results in hyperkalemia, hyponatremia, hypochloremia and acidemia by alterating reabsorption and secretion at the distal renal tubules.
iv. Urethral obstruction; ruptured bladder; anuric or oliguric renal failure; trichuriasis; salmonellosis; perforated duodenal ulcer; chylothorax with repeated drainage; tumor lysis syndrome; reperfusion of extremities after aortic thromboembolism in cats; insulin deficiency; non-specific beta blockers; drugs such as angiotensin-converting enzyme inhibitors, potassium sparing diuretics, NSAIDs and heparin therapy; metabolic acidosis due to mineral acids; thrombocytosis.
v. 0.2 units/kg regular insulin i/v followed by 2 grams dextrose/unit of insulin + 2.5% dextrose CRI; or calcium gluconate i/v; or 10% dextrose or 0.25 ml/kg 50% dextrose i/v. Give sodium bicarbonate (1–2 mmol/kg) if acidemic.

61 i. Pyometra, based on history, clinical signs, leukocytosis and purulent vaginal discharge.
ii. Pyometra occurs during diestrus when progesterone secretion is maximal. Animals which have received hormonal therapy are at increased risk of developing uterine infections.
iii. The definitive treatment for pyometra is ovariohysterectomy. This dog is dehydrated and azotemic and should be treated aggressively with bactericidal antibiotics and i/v fluids before anesthesia. Medical therapy could be considered in this dog if the owners desire future breeding, since she is a young dog with an open pyometra. Hospitalization and supportive care are combined with the administration of prostaglandin therapy (0.25 mg/kg s/c every 24 hours for 5 days) and systemic bactericidal antibiotics. Antibiotic therapy should be continued for 3–4 weeks. A second 5-day course of prostaglandin treatment may be required if the vaginal discharge is still present after 2 weeks. The bitch should be bred at the next estrus. The risk of uterine rupture and peritonitis is greater with medical therapy than with ovariohysterectomy.
iv. This bitch is azotemic and dehydrated but the urine is not concentrated. In pyometra the inability to concentrate urine is usually the result of *E. coli* endotoxins inhibiting water reabsorption by renal collecting ducts. The bitches commonly have an obligatory polyuria and compensatory polydypsia. Proteinuria is common and may be associated with a urinary tract infection or glomerulonephritis. Prerenal azotemia should improve with rehydration.

62–64: Questions

62 A two-year-old, spayed female domestic shorthair cat fell eight floors about 30 minutes ago (**62**). She is bleeding from the mouth, shows labored respirations and is slightly depressed. She has pale mucous membranes and a delayed pupillary light response, both direct and consensual. She is able to stand but not to walk. Her CRT is >3 seconds and she has weak femoral pulses. Her lungs can not be heard on the right side and there are moist crackles on the left side. She

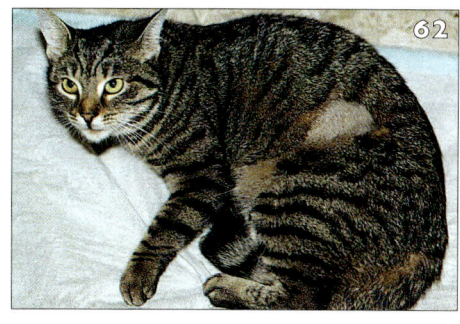

has a dysynchronous (choppy) movement of the chest and abdomen, with an abdominal component to her breathing. HR – 160 bpm; RR – 60 bpm; temperature – 97.9°F (36.6°C).
i. How would you characterize the cat's perfusion?
ii. List, in order of priority, the problems for this cat.
iii. List with priority your diagnostic, therapeutic and monitoring plans.
iv. The cat stabilizes, but after 40 minutes the breathing becomes labored again. What do you do now?

63 This dog (**63**) was hit by a car 60 minutes prior to presentation. He is showing signs of shock. On examination, circular bruising is noted around the umbilicus.
i. What does the bruising most likely indicate?
ii. Name two therapeutic procedures that can be used to stabilize intra-abdominal hemorrhage prior to performing surgery.

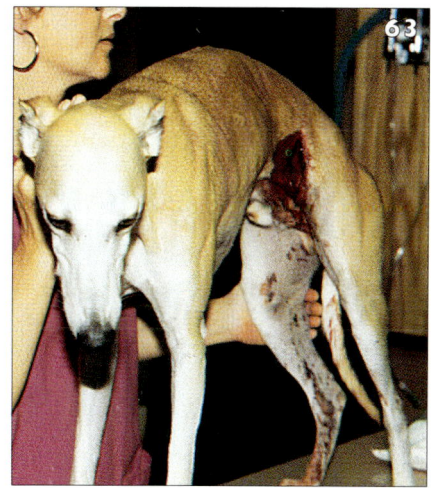

64 i. What are the benefits of pre-emptive (preprocedure) analgesia?
ii. What are the pros and cons of the following postoperative pain control medications in the critical patient: i/v butorphanol; i/v oxymorphone; i/v acepromazine; epidural morphine; local lidocaine.

62–64: Answers

62 i. The cat is in the middle (early decompensatory) stage of shock.
ii. Poor perfusion – weak pulses, prolonged CRT, pale gums; labored breathing with no lung sounds heard on right, moist on left; head trauma – delayed eye reflexes and mental depression; inability to walk.
iii. Therapeutic plan: flow-by oxygen; i/v catheter – balanced isotonic crystalloid (50 ml quickly, but as little as possible to resuscitate to protect the brain from cerebral edema; thoracocentesis left side chest; after fluids, 5 ml/kg hydroxyethyl starch over 5–10 minutes to increase BP, but maintaining systolic pressure slightly hypotensive (i.e. 80–100 mmHg); analgesics such as butorphanol; keep head elevated, do not use jugular veins, keep head position normal. Monitoring plan: BP – employ hypotensive resuscitation; ECG; PCV/TS for blood loss; blood gases (especially CO_2) to establish need for ventilation; repeat neurologic evaluation. Diagnostic plan: emergency data base: PCV, TS, dextrose, BUN, sodium, potassium; CBC, chemistry profile, urinalysis when stable; radiographs of chest and abdomen with pelvis, when stable; blood gases; neurologic examination.
iv. Tap chest and evacuate any air. If there is more pleural air, place a chest tube, apply continuous suction and re-evaluate breathing pattern and effort. If there is no air, then sedate the cat, intubate and ventilate.

63 i. Intra-abdominal hemorrhage. The bruising results from seepage of RBCs through a small umbilical defect.
ii. External abdominal counterpressure and internal abdominal counterpressure, the latter by the infusion of up to 20 ml/kg of crystalloids into the peritoneal space to provide an internal tamponading effect.

64 i. Benefits include a relatively pain-free procedure with less anesthetic required, and more effective post-procedure pain control with less postoperative medication required.
ii. Pros and cons of pain control medications in the critical patient are given in the table.

Agent	Pros	Cons
I/v butorphanol	Less respiratory and cardiac depression Good analgesic	Not quite as potent as agonists
I/v oxymorphone	Does not initiate histamine release Potent analgesic Reversible	Auditory hypersensitivity May cause bradycardia May cause hypotension May cause panting Controlled substance
I/v acepromazine	Potentiates analgesic agents Provides muscle relaxation	Enhances sedation Can be hypotensive
Epidural morphine	Prolonged analgesia Decreases amount of intra- and postoperative analgesia required	Can cause respiratory depression and hypotension if injected into the subarachnoid space Requires 30–40 minutes for complete effect May cause splanchnic vasodilation and urinary retention
Local lidocaine	Good local anesthesia Systemic anesthesia not required	Painful on injection

65 & 66: Questions

65 A ten-year-old, spayed female Boxer presents for evaluation of a collapsing episode lasting approximately 15 seconds in which she did not appear to be responsive. Past history revealed she had

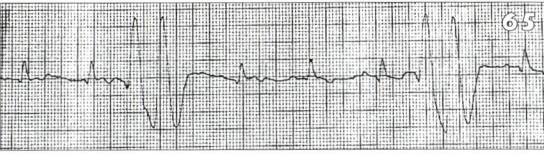

had three similar episodes within the last month. No abnormalities were detected on physical examination.
i. What is the ECG diagnosis (65) and what are your differentials at this point?
ii. What tests could be performed to confirm your suspicions?
iii. At what ventricular rate would it be unlikely that an arrhythmia is causing the hemodynamic trouble in the dog?

66 This 30 kg dog was hit by a car 30 minutes ago (66). Primary survey revealed: pale gum color with a CRT of 3 seconds; HR – 160 bpm; RR – 45 bpm; weak femoral pulses with absent dorsal metatarsal pulses. Initial data base: PCV – 55%; TS – 4.0 g/dl.
i. What stage of shock (compensatory, early decompensatory, decompensatory) is this patient in?
ii. List your initial plan for resuscitation. Include your fluid selection and why; rate of fluid administration; how you would monitor this patient.
iii. The following parameters are obtained while monitoring this patient. Explain what is happening, how you determined this from the data, and give your therapeutic intervention.

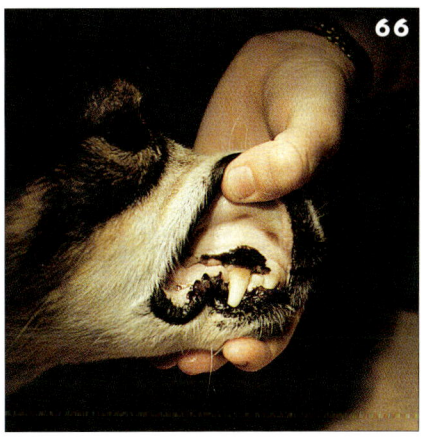

Time	PCV(%)/TS(g/dl)	HR (bpm)	BP (mmHg)	CVP
Initial	55/4.0	160	80/60	Not available
One hour later	35/3.2	140	150/80	Not available
Two hours later	22/2.1	188	68/45	2 cmH$_2$O

iv. The patient continues to decline. You have determined that the cause of the decompensation is occurring in the abdominal cavity. What is your plan of action?

65 & 66: Answers

65 i. Underlying rhythm is sinus at a ventricular rate of 140 bpm with VPCs in couplets. Boxer cardiomyopathy is probable.
ii. The difficulty arises in documenting the arrhythmia as these dogs often have a sinus tachycardia due to excitement or sinus arrhythmia on examination. A Holter recording may be necessary to document the heart rhythm during the syncopal episodes, especially if they occur infrequently. However, one should have strong suspicion if occasional ventricular ectopic beats are present.
iii. Between 80 and 120 bpm.

66 i. Early decompensatory shock.
ii. Initial fluid resuscitation should include an isotonic crystalloid infusion of a replacement solution at an initial rate of 40–90 ml/kg/hour. This can be combined with a colloid at 10–20 ml/kg while decreasing the amount of crystalloid infused by 40–60%. This dose may be decreased or increased depending on the patient's response (resuscitate only to a MAP of 80 mmHg [10.6 kPa]). Monitoring should include serial heart/pulse rates, mucous membrane color and CRT checks, pulmonary auscultation for moist lung sounds, and BP. In addition, CVP measurements and urine output measurements are ideal to determine the need for more or less intravascular volume. Serial PCV/TS measurements will suggest continuing blood loss and hemodilution.
iii. The initial PCV/TS findings suggest hemorrhage. Dogs can have splenic contraction that increases PCV and misleads the clinician into believing there is no hemorrhage. The low initial TS is a marker for hemorrhage in this case. The increased HR and decreased BP suggest shock, as explained above.

After initial fluid resuscitation the HR has decreased somewhat and the BP increased, indicating a response to fluid resuscitation. The PCV/TS levels have decreased, probably as a result of blood loss and hemodilution due to fluid infusion.

The 2 hour HR has dramatically increased and the BP dropped again. The concern is that there is low circulating volume as suggested by the low CVP, despite fluid volume. This indicates a worsening of the shock state, with ongoing hemorrhage.
iv. Abdominal counterpressure and hindlimb binding may decrease the flow of hemorrhage while the animal is prepared for surgery and a blood transfusion is being administered.

67 & 68: Questions

67 An eight-year-old mixed-breed dog is presented for a history of shaking and weakness. The owner notes that the dog has recently started to urinate in the house. The dog is pot-bellied and has a thin hair coat with no hair on the abdomen. The dog is panting heavily and the whole body is shaking. No pain can be localized and the dog collapses when pressure is put on its back. Hematology is as follows: segmented neutrophils – 30,375;

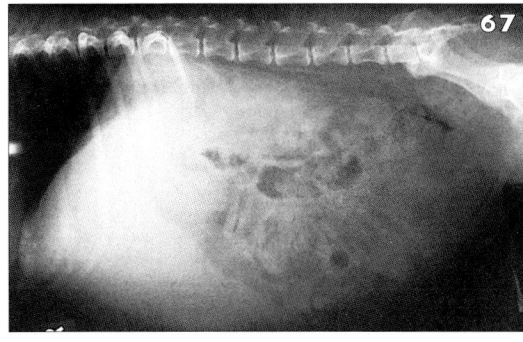

bands – 375; lymphocytes – 750; monocytes – 4000. ALT – 182 U/l; SAP – 2311 U/l; cholesterol – 304 mg/dl (7.9 mmol/l). Urinalysis: SG – 1.012 with sediment, 3+ proteinuria, 3–4 WBCs/hpf, 1–2 RBCs/hpf.
i. What is your differential diagnosis based on this information?
ii. The polyuria associated with hyperadrenocorticism is due to all of the following except for:
a. Interference with antidiuretic hormone.
b. Increased glomerular filtration rate.
c. Decreased release of vasopressin.
d. Increased level of aldosterone.
iii. The dog has a BP of 180/100 mmHg (24.0/13.3 kPa). What is the mechanism of this hypertension?

68 A two-year-old Labrador arrives after having been hit by a car. The owner reports the dog took his last breath in the parking lot. The dog is immediately intubated and ventilated with 100% oxygen. A moderate amount of blood is noted in the trachea during intubation.
i. During artificial ventilation with an AMBU bag you notice increasing resistance to ventilation. What is the most likely cause? What is the treatment? Be specific as to how you would treat this on an immediate basis.
ii. An ECG shows a fibrillatory rhythm. Due to his injuries and his size you decide the dog needs open chest CPR. Describe the technique for a rapid entry thoracotomy. Is clipping required?
iii. What vessels will most likely be cut near the sternum during this process, and what should be done about it?
iv. If you need a larger incision, what can be done?
v. Before starting cardiac compressions what should be done to the pericardium, and how?
vi. Compression of the aorta by cross-clamping is indicated during initial resuscitation. What is this, why is it done, and how is it done? How long can the clamp be safely left on?
vii. You have not been able to place a peripheral catheter due to poor pressure. What option(s) do you have for vascular access and how is this performed?

67 & 68: Answers

67 i. Cushing's disease and liver disease.
ii. d.
iii. There is enhanced reabsorption of sodium in the renal tubule due to the excessive cortisol. This results in secondary fluid retention and increased blood volume.

68 i. The dog probably has a tension pneumothorax. Treatment is an immediate minithoracotomy. A needle thoracocentesis will not be very effective in this case because air would be evacuated too slowly.
ii. Clipping is not required due to the time taken to perform this task. An incision is made at the 5th intercostal space on the left side from near the costovertebral junction to the sternum. A pair of curved Mayo scissors are then used to puncture in a controlled fashion into the pleural space. The blades are opened to allow air in and partially collapse the lung. With the blades partially open a pushing motion is used in a dorsal and ventral direction to separate all the layers of the thoracic musculature. Balfours are then placed in the incision.

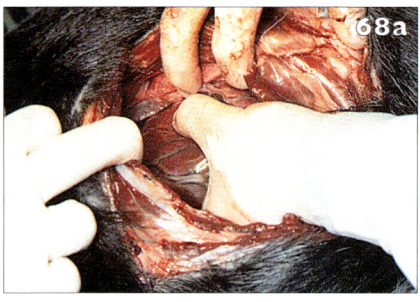
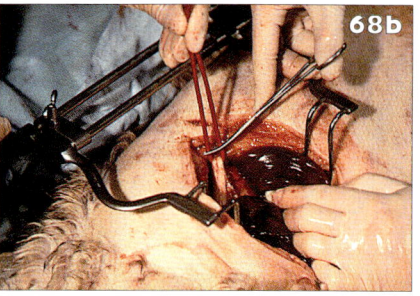

iii. The internal thoracic artery and vein can be transected. Once blood pressure returns, these vessels will start to bleed and will need to be ligated.
iv. The ribs on either side of the incision can be 'shingled'. This involves cutting the costochondral junctions and pushing the rib underneath the one beside it, thus creating a wider opening.
v. Cardiac compressions have been shown to be more effective if the pericardium is opened (**68a**). The sternopericardial ligament is hooked with the forefinger of the left hand. Using Mayo scissors, the pericardium is incised near the apex. The scissors are then used in a pushing action to open the pericardium, being careful to avoid the phrenic nerve.
vi. Cross-clamping is the placing of a clamp across the aorta to prevent arterial flow caudal to the thorax. The goal is to help improve cerebral circulation. Initially, digital pressure can be used to compress the descending thoracic aorta. Cross-clamping involves placing a vascular clamp or Rommel tourniquet around the descending aorta. A red rubber tube can be used if vascular clamps are not available (**68b**). The tube is passed around the aorta using blunt dissection and hemostats are used to clamp the ends of the tube together adjacent to the aorta, thus occluding the vessel. The aorta should not be clamped for longer than 10 minutes.
vii. A cutdown can be performed over a peripheral or central vessel. A large bore catheter can also be placed in the heart through an incision in the right auricle. A purse-string suture may need to be placed in the auricle prior to placing a stab incision. The tube is passed through the stab incision and the purse-string suture tightened.

69 & 70: Questions

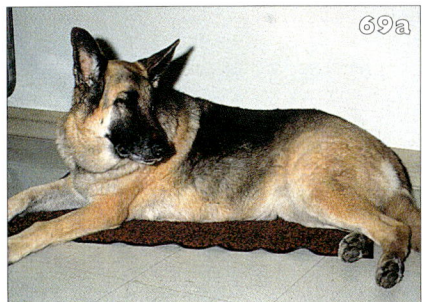
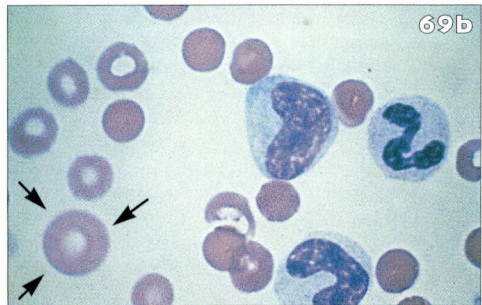

69 This six-year-old, spayed female German Shepherd Dog was presented for evaluation of lethargy of 3 days' duration (**69a**). Physical examination revealed pale mucous membranes, weakness and tachycardia. PCV – 12%, TS – 7.2 mg/dl; 30,000 reticulocytes.
i. Is the anemia in this patient regenerative or non-regenerative?
ii. List four differentials for the anemia in this patient.
iii. What is the abnormal erythrocyte morphology indicated by the arrows (**69b**)?
iv. Given this morphologic change in the RBCs, what is your primary differential diagnosis for the cause of the anemia in this dog.
v. What further diagnostic tests would you perform to confirm your diagnosis?

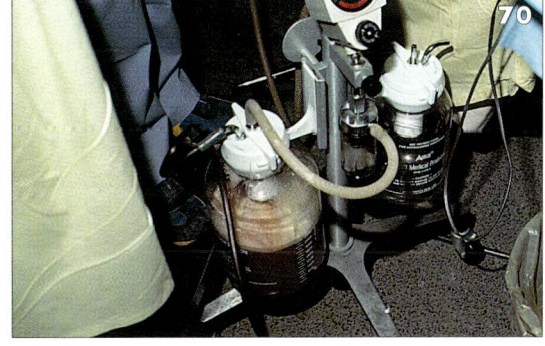

70 A dog that had been hit by a car is presented to your hospital. The dog had both a hemoabdomen and a hemothorax, and now has a PCV of 15%. There is no blood available for transfusion and so you have decided to autotransfuse (**70**).
i. What is autotransfusion?
ii. In the case of acute hemorrhage, blood from the thorax is ideal for three reasons. What are they?
iii. What is the major concern with autotransfusing blood from the abdominal cavity?
iv. What is the major complication of autotransfusion?
v. If blood is collected within the first few hours of hemorrhage, does anticoagulant need to be added to blood from the pleural cavity or peritoneal cavity?
   A filter is not available. The patient's PCV is 17%; TS is 3.0 g/dl. No other blood products are available.
vi. Why should or should not the blood be given?

69 & 70: Answers

69 i. Non-regenerative. By definition, a regenerative anemia is present when the corrected reticulocyte count is >60,000.
ii. Acute hemorrhage or hemolysis (before RBC regeneration occurs); iron deficiency; myeloproliferative disease; or chronic disease such as hypothyroidism, chronic renal failure or neoplasia.
iii. Spherocytes.
iv. The primary differential for anemia with spherocytes is IMHA. Although not specific for primary or secondary immune-mediated destruction, spherocytosis is the hallmark of IMHA.
v. Slide agglutination and Coombs' tests, and bone marrow aspiration. Bone marrow aspiration may aid in the diagnosis of IMHA. In dogs with IMHA the bone marrow is typically active with increased cellularity and a normal to decreased myeloid:erythroid ratio. Erythroid hyperplasia with or without hyperplasia of the myeloid and/or megakaryocytic cell lines is the most common finding. Erythrophagocytosis or agglutination of erythroid precursors may indicate an immunologic mechanism of anemia.

70 i. The process of reinfusing blood retrieved from bleeding cavities back into the patient.
ii. No anticoagulant is needed; blood is usually not contaminated; removal of blood is therapeutic.
iii. Contamination from intestinal contents if the bowel is ruptured.
iv. Disseminated intravascular coagulation.
v. If blood is being used for autotransfusion, the addition of anticoagulant is always safer and is always required for blood retrieved from the abdomen. However, if retrieved from the thorax within the first few hours and rapidly reinfused into the patient, autotransfused blood does not require anticoagulant.
vi. Blood should be given if the patient is in a critical condition, as survival has been reported when blood is given without the use of a filter in life-threatening circumstances.

71 & 72: Questions

71 A three-year-old, intact male Great Dane is presented with mild depression and anorexia (71a). The dog lives outside on a farm. Physical examination reveals: HR – 160 bpm; mucous membranes - bright pink; CRT – 1 second; femoral pulses – bounding; swollen muzzle; and tissue swelling on the neck, ventral to the lower jaw, approximately 8 inches (20 cm) in diameter.
i. What are the most life-threatening problems in this dog?
ii. What are the most likely differential diagnoses?
iii. What is your diagnostic plan?
iv. What are your treatment and monitoring plans for viper snake bite?
v. Would you use antivenom, or not?

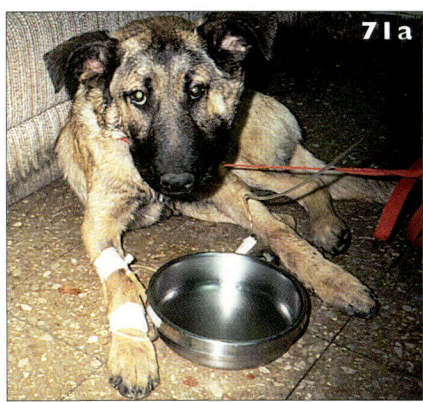

72 i. When attempting to control hemorrhage, vessels may need to be temporarily occluded. Match the following vessels with times of occlusion that can be safely performed without compromising organ function:

Ascending aorta	30 minutes
Descending thoracic aorta	15–20 minutes
Portal triad	10–15 minutes
Hepatic artery	30 minutes
Splenic artery and vein	2–3 minutes
Renal artery and vein	5–10 minutes
Abdominal aorta	30 minutes

ii. Occlusion times for some vessels may be prolonged when two events occur. What are they?
iii. To which of the above vessels does this not apply?
iv. Vascular clamps are often ideal for temporary occlusion of blood vessels. However, vascular loops can be created by placing loops of material around a vessel and tightening them. Name three materials that can be used to create 'vascular loops'.

71 & 72: Answers

71 i. The dog is in the compensatory stage of shock. The two main immediate concerns are possible progression to the decompensatory stages of shock and upper airway obstruction.

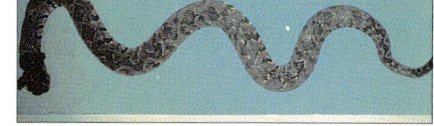

ii. The systemic and localized signs are most compatible with snake or insect bite. Less likely are hematoma, abscess, salivary obstruction, ruptured neoplasia, foreign body penetration or trauma.

iii. A thorough history should help if snake bite is suspected. Clipping the erythematous area of the swelling might expose fang or sting puncture wounds. Cytologic evaluation of fine needle aspirates, CBC and blood smear, and a coagulation profile may rule in or rule out the differential diagnoses.

iv. Viper (**71b**) toxins may cause hemolysis, neurotoxicity, cardiac dysrhythmias and tissue necrosis. The fangs are contaminated and may cause bacterial infection and local tissue necrosis. The treatment should consist of i/v crystalloids and colloids; oxygen support; blood products as needed; antibiotics effective against Gram-positive and Gram-negative aerobes and anaerobes; consider the use of antivenin. The use of glucocorticoids is controversial. Cardiac function and perfusion parameters must be monitored closely for a minimum of 24–48 hours, anticipating the complications seen in SIRS. In case of severe dyspnea due to upper airway obstruction, tracheotomy or endotracheal intubation should be performed and ventilation and oxygenation supported.

v. The use of antivenin depends on the type of snake, potency and amount of venom injected, size of the animal bitten, and severity of clinical signs. If vipers are common in your area, or if the owner identified it, adminster the specific antivenin after an intradermal skin test. Otherwise, a polyvalent antivenin can be used.

72 i.

Ascending aorta	2–3 minutes
Descending thoracic aorta	5–10 minutes
Portal triad	10–15 minutes
Hepatic artery	30 minutes
Splenic artery and vein	15–20 minutes
Renal artery and vein	30 minutes
Abdominal aorta	30 minutes

ii. Occlusion times can be prolonged if the patient is hypothermic or given shock doses of short-acting corticosteroids.
iii. The ascending aorta.
iv. Umbilical tape; Penrose drains; red rubber tubes or wide, sterile rubber bands.

73 & 74: Questions

73 A nine-year-old, castrated male Labrador Retriever presents on a hot summer's day with stridorous breathing and a temperature of 104°F (40°C). The owners have noted that lately the dog has seemed to tire early on walks. HR is 120 bpm with no auscultable murmurs or arrhythmias.
i. What is the most likely diagnosis, and how would you confirm this?
ii. The dog becomes more agitated in the examination room and begins to develop cyanotic mucous membranes. What procedures do you perform immediately?
iii. What specific set of diagnostic tests would be appropriate to determine whether there is an underlying cause for this condition?

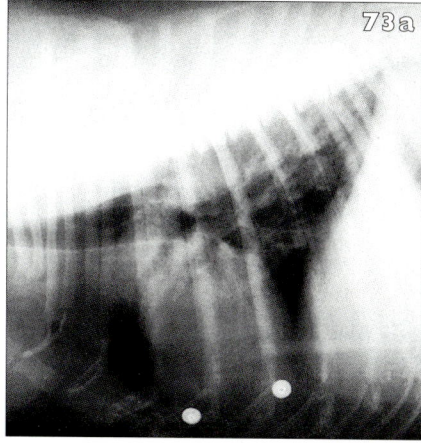

iv. What long-term therapeutic procedures would you recommend?
v. Once the dog has been stabilized and the inspiratory stridor has decreased, auscultation reveals mild and diffuse crackles on inspiration. Thoracic radiographs are shown (73a). How can you explain this pattern given your presumed diagnosis?

74 This four-year-old dog is presented for abdominal distension, rapidly progressive lethargy and non-productive retching (74).
i. What is your primary rule-out for this dog?
ii. Prioritize the following therapeutic/diagnostic modalities which are important in the initial management of this patient. Which should be performed first and why?
a. ECG and correction of any arrhythmias seen.

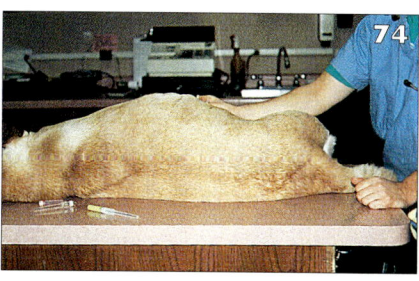

b. Abdominal radiographs to confirm suspected displacement of stomach.
c. Large bore i/v catheter placement and rapid i/v fluid administration.
d. Gastric decompression by tube placement or trocharization.
e. Administration of corticosteroids.
iii. True or false?: successful placement of an orogastric tube can rule out gastric volvulus and eliminate the need for radiographs or further therapy.

73 & 74: Answers

73 i. Laryngeal paralysis. Gentle pressure on laryngeal palpation may cause marked stridor, leading to a suspicion of laryngeal paralysis. Once the dog is stable, light sedation will allow visualization of the laryngeal arytenoid cartilages for abduction and evidence of edema (73b).

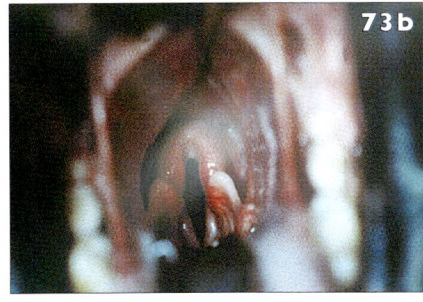

ii. Sedation with acepromazine (0.05 mg/kg i/v) should be considered, as well as supplementation of oxygen, i/v fluid support, corticosteroids (prednisolone sodium succinate [2–4 mg/kg i/v] or dexamethasone sodium phosphate [0.2–2.2 mg/kg i/v]). A transtracheal oxygen catheter may provide adequate oxygen concentrations during initial medical stabilization. Anesthesia and intubation may be necessary. Tracheostomy should be considered if extubation is not possible.

iii. A CBC and chemistry profile should be performed to evaluate for systemic disease. Chest and cervical radiographs should be evaluated for masses (tumors, abscesses, granulomas, foreign bodies) which may be compressing the recurrent laryngeal nerve or causing physical impairment of laryngeal motion. The presence of a megaesophagus may be evident on thoracic radiographs. Because of the reported association of laryngeal paralysis with hypothyroidism and neuromuscular diseases (laryngeal paralysis-polyneuropathy complex), a TSH stimulation test, electromyography and nerve conduction velocity measurements are recommended.

iv. Medical management is sometimes rewarding. Exercise restriction, corticosteroids (prednisone – 0.25–0.5 mg/kg p/o bid) and a cool environment may prevent the occurrence of dyspnea. Surgical options include partial arytenoidectomy, arytenoid lateralization and the castellated laryngofissure technique.

v. The mixed interstitial and alveolar infiltrates in the dorsocaudal lung fields in this radiograph are suggestive of non-cardiogenic pulmonary edema secondary to upper airway obstruction.

74 i. Gastric dilatation/volvulus
ii. c, e, a, d, b.
iii. False.

75–77: Questions

75 i. What factors determine central venous pressure (CVP) (75)?
ii. Does CVP measure circulatory volume?
iii. What is the proper placement for the catheter used for measuring CVP, and what is the ideal CVP measurement?

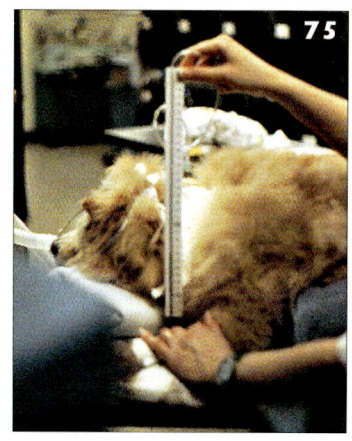

76 This two-year-old, castrated male domestic shorthair cat is presented with a 3-week history of progressive dyspnea, anorexia and occasional coughing. He is markedly more distressed today. HR – 160 bpm; RR – 45 bpm; temperature – 102.4°F (39.1°C). The cat has a dysynchrous, 'choppy' breathing pattern. On auscultation there are increased bronchovesicular sounds heard bilaterally in the dorsal lung fields, but the cranial lung fields are dull. His anterior thorax is non-compressible.
i. How do you initially stabilize the cat's condition?
ii. A thoracic radiograph is provided post thoracentesis (76). What is the diagnosis?
iii. How would you proceed to further characterize this finding?

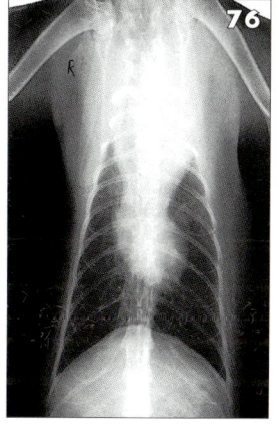

77 A seven-year-old, neutered male German Shepherd Dog collapsed during his morning walk. There was a 2–3 day history of lethargy and mild weakness, and no possibility of trauma. Initial physical examination revealed pale mucous membranes; CRT – 3 seconds; HR – 160 bpm; weak femoral pulses and no dorsal metatarsal pulses; temperature – 100.4°F (38°C). Abdominal palpation revealed a fluid wave and an enlarged spleen with a very globular, irregular surface. The heart sounds were muffled and there was jugular distension. Initial laboratory results were: PCV – 35%; TS – 5.0 g/dl; BUN – 11 mg/dl; glucose – 60 mg/dl (3.3mmol/l). There was moderate fluid distension in the abdomen.
i. What differential diagnosis is considered for this animal?
ii. What diagnostics would you pursue at this time?
iii. What cardiac abnormalities are anticipated in this animal?
iv. What coagulation abnormality is anticipated with the problems of this dog?
v. What is the long-term prognosis for the malignant form of this splenic problem?

75–77: Answers

75 i. Hydrostatic pressure in the vena cava, which is a function of right heart function, venous distensibility, intrathoracic pressure and central venomotor activity.
ii. No. However, changes in CVP may reflect changes in circulatory volume.
iii. The tip of the catheter used for measuring CVP should ideally be at the heart base, just proximal to the right atrium. The ideal CVP in a normal animal is between –1 and 5 cmH_2O, and 2–8 cmH_2O in the critically ill patient.

76 i. Oxygen supplementation should be initiated. Because the lack of lung sounds in the ventral thorax is consistent with pleural fluid, thoracocentesis is indicated. If a mediastinal mass is suspected, corticosteroids may improve ventilation by decreasing the mass size and reducing tracheal inflammation at the sight of compression. However, if the cat is stable, corticosteroids and chemotherapy should be withheld until diagnostic cytology has been performed.
ii. A mediastinal mass.
iii. The differential diagnoses for mediastinal masses in cats include lymphosarcoma (of which 80% occur in FeLV positive cats), thymoma, thyroid adenocarcinoma, abscess and granuloma. Additional diagnostic approaches would include pleural fluid analysis, FeLV test and a fine-needle aspirate or ultrasound-guided biopsy of the mass. Consider a coagulation profile before biopsy.

77 i. Hemangioma, hemangiosarcoma, hematoma of the spleen, splenic torsion, other splenic tumors, splenic nodular hyperplasia.
ii. Abdominal and thoracic radiographs; abdominal ultrasound examining the spleen and liver for evidence of lesions; cardiac echo for evaluation for right atrial mass or pericardial effusion; CBC, chemistry profile, urinalysis; coagulation profile with platelet count; abdominocentesis with ultrasound and fluid analysis.
iii. Pericardial effusion and ventricular ectopic beats.
iv. Acute or chronic disseminated intravascular coagulation is likely due to the exposure of subendothelial collagen and release of tissue thromboplastin from the damaged splenic tissues.
v. Survival times for hemangiosarcoma: median survival times for surgery alone range from 19 to 65 days. Median survival time in 15 dogs with chemotherapy and splenectomy was 172 days.

78–80: Questions

78 A five-year-old, female St Bernard (80 kg) is presented for a sudden onset of vomiting. The dog is still walking normally and is bright and alert. The owner says that the dog has vomited five times in the last hour and the vomitus is white and thick. Physical examination reveals bright pink mucous membranes; CRT – <2 seconds; HR – 150 bpm; RR – 30 bpm; bounding femoral pulses; dorsal metatarsal pulses present. Abdominal palpation reveals some tightness in the cranial

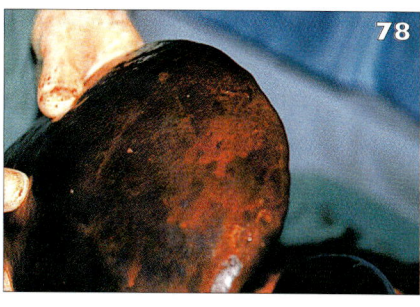

abdomen but it is difficult to palpate structures clearly due to the massive size of the dog. Abdominal radiographs show a greatly enlarged spleen, displaced dorsally and to the right. The stomach appears to be of normal size and in the normal position. This was confirmed by a contrast study of the stomach. The spleen on this second set of films is now larger than it was on the survey radiographs and appears to have a 'C' shape.
i. What is the most likely diagnosis?
ii. Outline your initial preoperative management.
iii. How many milliliters of crystalloid would this dog receive in the first hour if 'shock rate' crystalloids were given? What are your concerns about resuscitating with crystalloids alone?
iv. Outline your intraoperative concerns at the time of surgical management of this case.
v. What postoperative complications might you expect in this patient?

79 A nine-year-old, castrated male Golden Retriever (40 kg) presents with an acute onset of exercise intolerance following a walk. He is unable to stand, tachypneic, the heart is difficult to auscultate and pulsus paradoxus are noted.
i. What other abnormalities might your examination reveal in this patient?
ii. What is pulsus paradoxus?
iii. What radiographic (79) and ECG findings might be present?
iv. What is cardiac tamponade, and how would you diagnose it?
v. How much pericardial effusion is significant, and what would be appropriate immediate interventions?

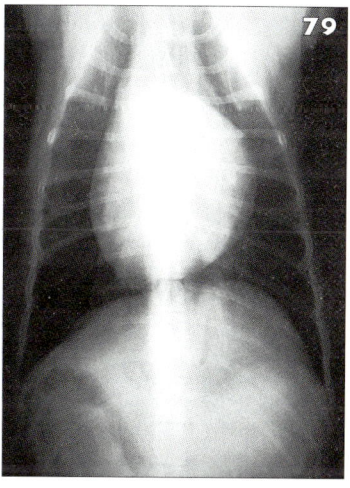

80 A cat with cerebral trauma is presented for repair of an open fracture of the humerus. What would be your principal concerns for managing the head injury during anesthesia in this patient?

78–80: Answers

78 i. Splenic torsion (though splenic tumor or hematoma is possible).
ii. Begin i/v fluids utilizing a combination of crystalloids and colloids. Blood loss in this dog will quite possibly be substantial due to trapping of blood in the spleen. The dog is likely to need blood. A transfusion from a donor dog can be initiated and autotransfusion utilized if additional blood products are required. The dog should receive oxygen and analgesics. His ECG should be evaluated as should his PCV, TS, glucose, BUN, electrolytes, ACT and platelets.
iii. 80 kg × 90 ml/kg = 7200 ml of crystalloids in the first hour. Concerns about utilizing crystalloids alone include the increase time required to administer 7 liters, the dilution of oncotic proteins, and the likelihood that the fluid will extravasate into the lungs, spleen and abdomen.
iv. The dog's spleen at the time of surgery is shown (78). Concerns include: do not untwist the spleen; assessing for thrombosis of splenic vessels and deciding whether or not a total or partial splenectomy is required; engorged spleens are easily ruptured and require careful handling; preservation of the left gastroepiploic artery is ideal; careful ligation of the short gastric vessels which could potentially cause gastric necrosis.
v. Hemorrhage from inadequate splenic vessel ligation; hypovolemia and anemia due to sequestered blood loss; endotoxemia due to ischemia and vascular stasis; inflammatory response syndrome, with arrhythmias and DIC.

79 i. Tachycardia, jugular venous distension and ascites.
ii. Pulsus paradoxus is a large drop (>10 mmHg) in systolic blood pressure with inspiration, called paradoxical because of the disappearance of the pulse during inspiration when the heart is obviously still beating.
iii. The chest radiograph usually demonstrates an enlarged cardiac silhouette with clear lung fields. The cardiac silhouette may not be enlarged in an acute situation. The ECG may have electrical alternans or low QRS voltage and T-wave flattening.
iv. Cardiac tamponade occurs when the atria and ventricles are prevented from filling adequately due to excess pericardial effusion. This reduces stroke volume and causes hemodynamic compromise.
v. In a dog this size, acutely – 100–200 ml; chronically – up to 1500 ml. An immediate pericardiocentesis should be performed once effusion is confirmed and cardiac tamponade is present. Stabilization also includes i/v fluid therapy for volume expansion to prevent diastolic collapse of the heart.

80
- Ensure adequate circulation and oxygen supply. Do not allow hypotension or hypertension.
- Ensure adequate analgesia with agents such as butorphanol/diazepam or oxymorphone/diazepam.
- Prevent hypertension - avoid ketamine.
- Do not allow coughing or sneezing during intubation or extubation since this can increase intracranial pressure. Administration of lidocaine prior to intubation can offset these signs.
- Ensure that arterial PCO_2 is between 30 and 35 mmHg (4.0 and 6.7 kPa).
- Ensure that the head is level with the body or elevated no more than 20 degrees. Make sure that the head is never below the body.
- The head should be maintained at a normal 45 degree angle to the body.
- Avoid occluding the jugular veins.

81–83: Questions

81 A four-year-old crossbred dog is presented with sudden onset bilateral blindness. The owner had exercised the dog regularly and was quite certain that all sight had been lost over a 48 hour period. There was no indication of ocular pain and examination demonstrated bilateral mydriasis. Both the direct and consensual light reflexes were absent. The cornea and lens were transparent and the appearance of the fundus was as depicted (81).
i. What is the differential diagnosis?
ii. What is SARD, and what is the suggested cause?
iii. What treatment can you prescribe?

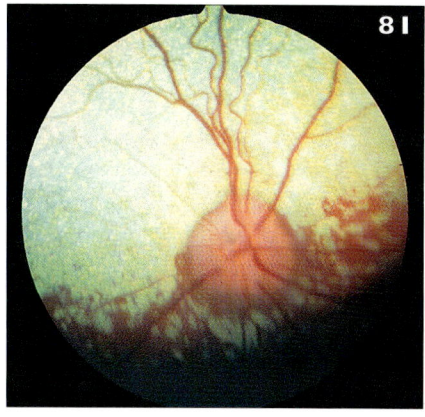

82 A four-year-old, castrated male German Shorthaired Pointer presented with a severe necrotizing fasciitis/cellulitis of the ventral thoracic wall. Two days into treatment following resection of the involved area the dog developed tachypnea and an increased ventilatory effort. Thoracic radiographs were taken; the lateral view is shown (82).
i. What is the most likely diagnosis of these radiographic changes?
ii. What is the likely pathophysiologic process that led to these changes?
iii. How is this condition diagnosed?
iv. How is this condition treated?
v. What criteria would indicate the need for mechanical ventilation in this patient?
vi. What monitoring should be employed in this patient?

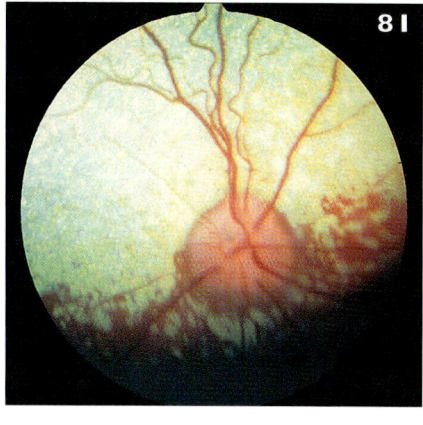

83 A 13-year-old, castrated male mixed terrier was presented with a 3-day history of anorexia with 1 day of multiple episodes of vomiting. The owner reported that the dog had previously been diagnosed with chronic renal disease and was currently being managed at home with low protein diet, phosphate binders and s/c fluids. The dog was underweight with some muscle atrophy. Dehydration based on dry mucus membranes and decreased skin turgor was estimated to be 4–5%. There was a severe malodor to the breath. The kidneys were small, smooth and non-painful. Melanic stool was found on rectal examination.
PCV – 29%; TS – 7.8 g/dl; BUN – 120 mg/dl; creatinine – 4.2 mg/dl (371.3 µmol/l); phosphorus – 4.7 mg/dl. A urine dipstick test of the vomitus was positive for occult blood.
i. What is the most likely cause of vomiting and GI tract bleeding in this dog?
ii. Which of the following would be the best initial therapy for uremic gastritis: ice water lavage; oral antacids administered bid; surgical excision; sucralfate administered 2–3 times per day; combination therapy with oral antacids and cimetidine?
iii. If this patient has persistent vomiting, which antiemetic would you add to the therapy and why?

81–83: Answers

81 i. The fundus appears normal. The loss of sight and the bilateral absence of both reflexes could indicate an optic nerve or optic tract lesion, but the possibility of SARD should be considered.
ii. SARD is due to a rapid loss of photoreceptor function; 'undetermined toxicity' has been the suggested cause.
iii. There is no treatment. Ophthalmoscopic examination will reveal progressive extensive retinal degeneration over the following 3–4 months.

82 i. Acute respiratory distress syndrome (ARDS).
ii. Lung injury secondary to endothelial damage, leading to increased pulmonary capillary permeability and pulmonary edema with a normal PCWP (indicates pulmonary vascular hydrostatic pressure). Endothelial damage may be caused directly (e.g. aspiration or bacterial pneumonia) or by inflammatory mediator activation.
iii. Criteria for diagnosis include hypoxemia, diffuse lung infiltrates on thoracic radiographs, decreased pulmonary compliance, increased ventilatory rate and normal PCWP.
iv. Treatment should be initiated for the inciting cause plus oxygen supplementation and other supportive care for the SIRS, e.g. nutritional, cardiovascular.
v. Criteria for mechanical ventilatory support in this patient include PaO_2 <60 mmHg (<8.0 kPa) and/or $PaCO_2$ >50 mmHg (>6.7 kPa) when patient is on supplemental oxygen. Mechanical ventilatory support is also provided if the patient's respiratory effort is increasing.
vi. Monitoring the pulmonary system would include arterial blood gases, thoracic radiographs, SaO_2, end-tidal CO_2, perfusion parameters and careful auscultation. Monitoring will need to be done also for other SIRS complications (e.g. coagulation profiles, ATIII, platelets to monitor for DIC) and to guide therapy. BP, HR, CVP and perfusion parameters for circulation and systemic perfusion.

83 i. Uremic gastritis due to increased gastrin-attenuated gastric mucosa and platelet dysfunction.
ii. Sucralfate administered 2–3 times per day.
iii. Vomiting associated with uremia has both central and peripheral components. Circulating uremic toxins initiate vomiting via stimulation of the chemoreceptor trigger zone (CMTZ) D_2-dopaminergic receptors, best controlled with metoclopramide. The peripheral component (uremic gastritis) is controlled with sucralfate and/or H_2-histaminergic antagonists such as cimetidine.

84–86: Questions

84 This radiograph (84) (Courtesy Dr P Wolvekamp) is from a four-year-old, male Scottish Sheepdog 2 hours after it was rescued from a burning house. When the dog was brought to the hospital it was dyspneic and had bright red mucous membranes. It also had signs of smoke inhalation, consisting of facial burns and soot-stained nasal discharge and saliva.

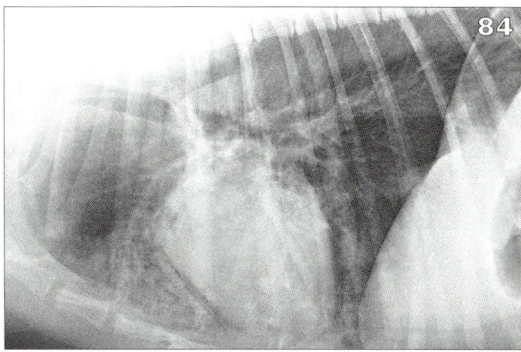

i. What are the two main causes of these radiographic changes?
ii. Can it be concluded from the appearance of the mucous membranes that the oxygen content of the blood is not severly diminished?
iii. How useful are blood gas analyses in this respect?
iv. What are the three main causes of tissue hypoxia after smoke inhalation?

85 Abdominal hemorrhage and a prolonged ACT were found in this seven-year-old Irish Setter 12 hours after exploratory surgery for septic peritonitis (85).
i. What laboratory tests would you use to confirm a diagnosis of DIC?
ii. How would you treat this patient?

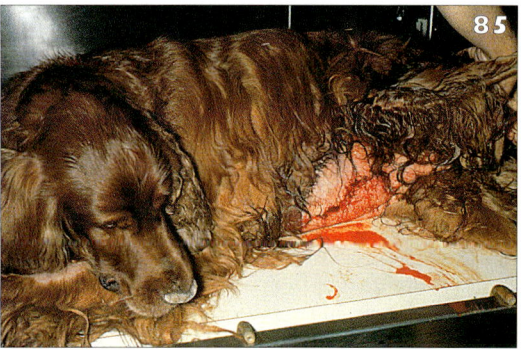

86 You are asked to advise a veterinary colleague on the importance of pre-emptive analgesia in companion animal patients.
i. Explain the philosophy behind pre-emptive analgesia.
ii. Explain the importance of pre-emptive analgesia.
iii. Explain the principles of pre-emptive analgesia.

84–86: Answers

84 i. There is both thermal and chemical damage to the respiratory tract. Thermal damage to the upper airways can cause suffocating laryngospasm, edema, hypersecretion and ulcerations. This leads to upper airway obstruction. Hot carbon particles can cause thermal damage to the lower airways. Chemical vapors (carbon monoxide, sulfur oxide, hydrogen chloride, hydrogen cyanide and aldehydes) can enter freely or attach to carbon particles and cause inactivation of ciliary movement and surfactant, with resultant edema and pneumonia.
ii. In smoke inhalation, poisoning with carbon monoxide has to be considered. Carbon monoxide combines with hemoglobin to form carboxyhemoglobin which has a bright red color. If high concentrations of carboxyhemoglobin are present, cyanosis may not be apparent.
iii. Blood gas analyses should be used with caution. PaO_2 is a reflection of oxygen dissolved in the plasma and not toal oxygen content. Carbon monoxide and oxygen react with the same group in the hemoglobin molecule and since the affinity of carbon monoxide is 200 times greater than that of oxygen, carboxyhemoglobin is incapable of carrying oxygen. As a result, oxygen saturation is reduced but PaO_2 can be normal in carbon-monoxide poisoning.
iv. Tissue hypoxia can be the result of carbon monoxide poisoning, upper airway obstruction and diminished small airway patency.

85 i. Diagnostics useful in confirming the presence of DIC include platelet count, PTT, PT, ACT, measurement of FDPs, fibrinogen, and ATIII. The results of these tests vary with the severity and the longevity of the DIC.
ii. The successful management of DIC requires treatment of the underlying disease as well as treatment of all secondary conditions. The patient should be volume expanded to improve oxygen delivery to the tissues. Heparin therapy should be initiated to inhibit microvascular coagulation by activating antithrombin III. Recommended doses of heparin vary from 5–10 units/kg/hour i/v to complete therapeutic heparinization (150–600 units/kg/hour i/v). In dogs, heparin doses of 25–100 units/kg s/c tid to qid have been recommended. Because the anticoagulant activity of heparin is dependent on adequate serum levels of ATIII, low serum levels of ATIII should be supplemented via the administration of fresh whole blood or fresh-frozen plasma. Fresh whole blood t ransfusion will supply hemostatic levels of clotting factors as well as ATIII and RBCs.

86 i. The principle behind pre-emptive analgesia is that therapeutic measures are taken before pain occurs in the patient and not when the patient actually experiences pain.
ii. Achieving adequate analgesia before the pain (potentially) occurs prevents or minimizes the occurrence of pre- and postoperative pain hypersensitivity.
iii. When applying pre-emptive analgesia, adequate preoperative analgesia is (preferably) realized and adequate pain control is continued in the per- and postoperative phases. The focus is on prevention of initial development of pain hypersensitivity and minimizing chances for central hypersensitivity to be (re)initiated in a later phase of the treatment.

87 & 88: Questions

87 A two-year-old, 25 kg, entire male dog was referred for evaluation of intermittent vomiting of 5 days' duration, anorexia and progressive depression. On physical examination the dog was shaking and the mucous membranes were yellow/pink with a CRT of one second (87). The RR and pattern were normal, pulses were strong at 180/minute; rectal temperature was 103.1°F (39.5°C). Anterior abdominal pain was present; however, there was no organomegaly. The dog was estimated to be approximately 6% dehydrated. Abnormal

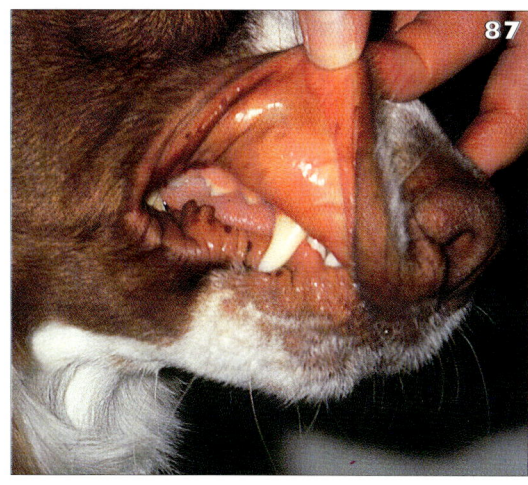

biochemical findings were conjugated bilirubin – 12.4 mg/dl (213 µmol/l); free bilirubin – 9.77 mg/dl (167 µmol/l); alkaline phosphatase – 866 U/l; GGT – 14 U/l; ALT – 4030 U/l; glucose – 54 mg/dl (3.0 mmol/l); urea – 41.5 mg/dl (6.9 mmol/l); creatinine – 0.6 mg/dl (56 µmol/l). Serum electrolytes were sodium – 157 mEq/l; potassium – 3.7 mEq/l; chloride – 115 mEq/l. While waiting further diagnostic procedures, the dog was placed on i/v fluids. Serum electrolytes at 8 hours were: sodium – 160 mEq/l; potassium – 3.9 mEq/l; chloride – 123 mEq/l. Urine output was considered normal, although not measured, with a SG of 1.023. The i/v fluid solution was changed. After 8 hours, the electrolytes were: sodium – 167 mEq/l; chloride – 125 mEq/l; potassium – 3.4 mEq/l. The i/v fluid solution was again changed. The dog became progressively oliguric with anuria occurring at 20 hours post admission.
i. Calculate a fluid plan, including type of solution, rate of delivery and electrolyte supplementation at initial presentation.
ii. What is your fluid of choice after receiving the second set of serum electrolytes?
iii. Explain the possible pathophysiologic events resulting in the rapidly occurring hypernatremia and anuria?
iv. How would you differentiate between the two possible events?

88 A four-week-old female Siamese kitten was found extremely depressed and unable to move. She was normal 6 hours previously. Physical examination: depressed mentation, temperature 99°F (37.3°C) and dry mucous membranes. Her gum color is gray and her femoral pulses weak. There are no external wounds and the abdomen palpates with fluid filled bowels. She is estimated to be 10% dehydrated. WBC count was 400/mm^3, primarily lymphocytes, and the glucose 40 mg/dl (2.24 mmol/l). The cat is FeLV and FIV negative. Fecal examination finds roundworms.
i. What is your immediate plan of action?
ii. You are unable to place an i/v catheter. What do you do, and how is it done?
iii. What fluid do you select?
iv. What is your working diagnosis, and what complications do you anticipate?

87 & 88: Answers

87 i. This dog is not in shock, therefore it is necessary to look at the rehydration plan. Six percent dehydration equals a fluid deficit of 0.06 × 25 kg = 1.5 liters. A temperature of 39.5°C is one degree above normal. For each degree Celsius above the normal of 38.5°C, add 10% of total daily fluid requirements: 10% of 1101 ml = 110 ml. Now add in the maintenance requirements for the 24 hour period. Maintenance volumes are normal ongoing losses which are divided into sensible and insensible losses. Sensible losses include water losses in urine and feces (which can be measured). The total volume of fluid to be administered during the first 24 hours is 1500 + 110 + 1101 = 2711 ml or 113 ml/hour. Any ongoing losses should be added. Isotonic alkalinizing solutions such as Plasma-Lyte 148^R, Normasol R^R or lactated Ringer's solution should be selected. 20 mEq/l) potassium and 50 ml 50% dextrose should be added to the i/v fluids (final dextrose concentration is 2.5%).
ii. Due to the rise in serum sodium, 2.5% dextrose in half-strength saline should replace the higher sodium-containing solutions above, once rehydrated.
iii. When urine output progressively diminishes in the presence of severe liver dysfunction, the hepatorenal syndrome should be considered. Hepatorenal syndrome occurs in the setting of both chronic and acute liver disease and an adequate intravascular volume. Diagnosis requires finding avid sodium retention, oliguria, hyposthenuria, absence of urinary obstruction and exclusion of intravascular volume depletion. Precipitating factors of hepatorenal syndrome include infections, large volume paracentesis, diarrhea, vomiting, nasogastric aspiration, contrast media, and drugs (NSAIDs, aminoglycosides). Volume depletion that causes prerenal azotemia and oliguria/anuria must be ruled out.
iv. Finding a urine creatinine:plasma creatinine ratio of >30 supports a diagnosis of hepatorenal syndrome; a ratio <30 suggests prerenal azotemia. The fractional excretion of sodium (F_ENa) can also be used to distinguish between the two. When the ratio is <1%, the hepatorenal syndrome is likely.

$$C_U/C_p > 30 \qquad \frac{(Na^+)_U \times (Creatine)_p}{(Na^+)_p \times (Creatine)_U} \times 100 = F_ENa$$

88 i. The animal has poor perfusion as well as dehydration. The perfusion must be corrected quickly with i/v fluids. The dehydration can be replaced over several hours. The fluid filled bowel suggests that the kitten is third body fluid spacing and will require more fluids than would be typically estimated. Warm the kitten once she is volume replaced. Give supplemental oxygen. Draw blood for data base and other laboratory tests. Give i/v or i/o crystalloids and colloids to re-establish perfusion and blood pressure over 15–30 minutes. Replace glucose with 0.5 g/kg i/v bolus and then supplement the fluids once able to provide maintenance fluids. Give i/v bactericidal antibiotics. Treat the roundworm infestation.
ii. The i/o route should be used (trochanteric fossa or greater tubercle of the humerus). Lidocaine is placed through the skin, subcutaneous tissue and periosteum. A 20G needle (spinal needle in mature animals) is inserted parallel to the long axis of the femur or humerus. The rate of administration is gradually increased over 5–10 minutes, reaching a typical maximum of 11 ml/minute.
iii. A balanced electrolyte solution, e.g. lactated Ringer's (intital rate 40 ml/kg/hour until perfusion has improved), will replace dehydration and part of the perfusion deficit. Hetastarch should be given (5 ml/kg over 10–20 minutes, repeated to desired effect).
iv. Feline panleukopenia. Complications include dehydration, diarrhea, sepsis, septic shock, hypoglycemia and malnutrition.

89 & 90: Questions

89 A four-year-old Golden Retriever presents in status epilepticus. History reveals that the dog has had intermittent seizure activity since 2 years of age. The frequency has been increasing over the past year, so the primary care veterinarian had placed the dog on oral phenobarbital. The dog had not seizured for over 4 months, so the owners discontinued the phenobarbital 2 days ago. The owners came home from a 2-hour excursion to find the dog in lateral recumbency, paddling, vocalizing and with evidence of urine and feces on the dog and on the floor. The dog made no signs of recognition when touched or when his name was called. Physical examination: temperature – 106°F (41.1°C); pulse – 180 bpm; RR – 38 bpm; mucous membranes – bright red; CRT – 1 second; pupil – dilated and non-responsive. The dog is still thrashing, paddling and vocalizing. Thoracic auscultation reveals primarily referred upper airway sounds, but the heart is synchronous with the pulse. The dog is estimated to be 8% dehydrated. Initial data base: PCV – 50%; TS – 8.0 g/dl; glucose labstick – 40 mg/dl (2.24 mmol/l); BUN labstick – 15–25 mg/dl; Na^+ – 145 mEq/l; K^+ – 4.2 mEq/l.

i. Comment on the time of onset of maximum action of the following agents given i/v: phenobarbital, pentobarbital, diazepam (**89**).
ii. List the problems that this dog has in order of priority.
iii. List your initial stabilization procedures in order of priority.
iv. Brain injury can occur secondarily to this prolonged seizure activity. Why?

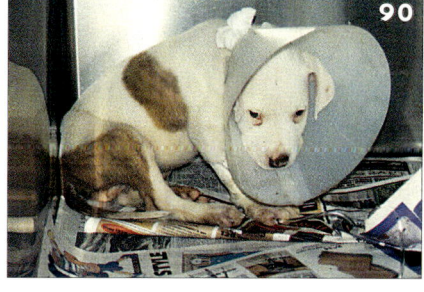

90 This three-month-old, unvaccinated Pit Bull Terrier (3 kg) presented for vomiting 12 times (clear to yellow foam) that day (**90**). He is severely depressed with a rectal temperature of 104°F (40°C). HR – 180 bpm; RR – 30 bpm; CRT – 2.5 seconds; mucous membranes gray and dry; normal skin turgor. Initial data base: PCV – 48%; TS – 5.0 g/dl; BUN – 40 mg/dl; glucose – 75 mg/dl (4.2 mmol/l).

i. In which fluid compartment(s) is the deficit in this dog (intravascular, interstitial, intracellular, or a combination)?
ii. Describe the effect of administration of the following fluids on each of the above fluid compartments in this patient: lactated Ringer's solution (LRS), 5% dextrose in water, hypertonic saline (7.5%), hetastarch, 5% dextrose in LRS.
iii. What is the best plan for replacing the fluid deficits you have identified in this dog with the least amount of fluids?
iv. Approximately 4 liters of LRS were administered to the dog over 18 hours. The dog is still dehydrated and has frequent vomiting and watery diarrhea. Explain the dehydration despite fluid administration, relating them back to the fluid compartments.

89 & 90: Answers

89 i. Phenobarbital – 30 minutes; pentobarbital – 5 minutes; diazepam – 8 minutes.
ii. Status epilepticus; hyperthermia; poor perfusion – tachycardia, red gums, rapid refill; hypoglycemia; dehydration; past history of seizures; sudden withdrawal of phenobarbital.
iii. Flow-by oxygen. Stop seizure activity: place i/v catheter and give pentobarbital to effect (until paddling slows); ideal plane is with no motor activity but good eye blink and ear twitch reflexes; the use of diazepam as the initial anticonvulsant in this severe, acute status epilepticus will likely produce ineffective or incomplete seizure control with early recurrent seizures; in addition, the combination of a barbiturate and diazepam causes greater respiratory depression than either agent used alone. Blood for data base and phenobarbital level and CBC and chemistry profile. I/v 50% glucose (0.5 g/kg). I/v crystalloids and consider colloids if poorly responsive blood pressure. Retake rectal temperature five minutes after seizures have stopped; if still elevated, place cool towels over dog until temperature is 103°F (39.4°C). Monitor blood glucose, neurologic status, urine output, ECG and BP. Pending serum phenobarbital levels, consider load dosing with phenobarbital once the dog begins waking up. Nursing care for the recumbent, head injured patient.
iv. Hypoxemia and hypotension; hypoglycemia, seizure activity and hyperthermia contribute to cerebral edema.

90 i. The intravascular and interstitial space.
ii. LRS will provide interstitial and partial intravascular fluid replacement. Hetastarch infusion will decrease the amount of fluid required for volume replacement. It appears also that oncotic support may be required as this patient is third spacing into the GI tract, in which case hetastarch would also be of benefit. Five percent dextrose in water will not adequately replace intravascular and interstitial space as it is a free-water replacement and will distribute into all compartments (two-thirds intracellular, one-third extracellular). Five percent dextrose in LRS will benefit this hypoglycemic patient after there has been interstitial fluid replacement. Using 5% dextrose in LRS or hypertonic saline in a dehydrated animal will cause fluid to move from the interstitium into the vascular space. If the patient is third spacing (e.g. a parvovirus patient) these fluids will quickly be unloaded from the intravascular space, exacerbating the dehydration.
iii. The best plan for fluid resuscitation would be a combination of isotonic crystalloid (such as LRS) and a colloid (such as hetastarch).
iv. Third spacing into the GI tract causes depletion of the intravascular fluid. The interstitial fluid is mobilized to replace acute intravascular fluid loss, causing dehydration. Diseased intestinal mucosa will also cause leakage of intravascular albumin, decreasing the fluid holding capacity of the intravascular space.

91–93: Questions

91 A six-year-old, castrated male, mixed-breed dog is presented with a 4-day history of vomiting and diarrhea. He presents in shock with a painful abdomen. You perform a needle abdominocentesis and retrieve a yellow-brown, turbid fluid. A cytologic preparation on a centrifuged sample of the fluid is shown (**91**).
i. What is your interpretation of the fluid sample?
ii. What therapy would you recommend based on this finding?
iii. Which of the following would be the best plan for initial fluid recuscitation for this patient.
a. I/v colloid at 20 ml/kg.
b. I/v crystalloid to replace the estimated dehydration deficit.
c. I/v colloid and crystalloid as needed to return perfusion parameters to normal.
d. Hypertonic saline at 8 ml/kg.
iv. You elect to use crystalloid. After administering the calculated fluid deficit, you observe no improvement in the dog's perfusion or hydration parameters. How do you explain this finding?
v. Name four other conditions where there may be significant third body spacing.
vi. Due to the difficulty in predicting the amount of fluid needed to maintain adequate perfusion and hydration in patients with a third body space fluid loss, describe the best method of monitoring fluid therapy in these patients.
vii. List five diagnostic findings in a vomiting patient with a distended painful abdomen that would be an absolute indication for surgical exploration.

92 An eight-year-old Golden Retriever is presented for acute collapse. The dog has pale mucous membranes and muffled heart sounds. The femoral pulses are weak. Thoracic radiographs show a globoid cardiac silhouette and increased interstitial densities in the lungs. An echocardiogram shows a hypoechoeic area between the heart and the pericardium, with restricted filling of the right and left ventricles during diastole.
i. What is the most likely cause of the acute collapse?
ii. What emergency procedure is required for stabilization of this dog and how is it safely performed?
iii. What is the reason for giving i/v fluids during this procedure?
iv. What other areas might be ultrasounded to aid in the diagnosis?

93 Your advice is sought in a case where a dog apparently has relapsed into stupor 24 hours after routine surgery and uneventful recovery.
i. What would be your first approach towards this patient?
ii. What is your differential diagnosis?
iii. What therapeutic measures would you consider?

91–93: Answers

91 i. Septic exudate with a mixed bacterial population. This finding suggests rupture or leakage of the GI tract.
ii. Abdominal exploration as soon as the dog can be stabilized for anesthesia.
iii. c.
iv. The peritoneal cavity is acting as a 'third body space'. Due to the regional inflammation, there is massive fluid leakage from the local interstitial and intravascular spaces.
v. Pyometra (uterus); severe diarrhea, e.g. parvovirus enteritis (GI tract); pancreatitis (peritoneal cavity); trauma (subcutaneous space).
vi. CVP (or capillary wedge pressure if available) and serial BP measurements.
vii. Radiographic evidence of free air; radiographic evidence of an obstruction secondary to a foreign body; demonstration of bilirubin in the abdominal fluid; demonstration of splenic or mesenteric torsion; evidence of rupture of the urinary tract.

92 i. Cardiac tamponade from pericardial effusion.
ii. Pericardiocentesis – the side to tap is determined by the thoracic radiograph. The chest wall is clipped and aseptically prepared between the 3rd and 9th intercostal spaces. Ideally, needle placement is guided with ultrasound. When ultrasound is not available, determine the rib space to enter from the DV thoracic radiographs. A flexible catheter with side holes is used for draining the pericardial fluid. An ECG is monitored for arrhythmias. The fluid is slowly removed and examined for PCV/TS and platelets, to differentiate it from whole blood from a cardiac puncture. If it is found to be whole blood, only remove enough fluid to relieve the life-threatening tamponade and then stop until the origin of the whole blood is determined (e.g. cardiac puncture with centesis, ruptured atrium, bleeding mass).
iii. When the pressure on the ventricles caused by the pericardial fluid is relieved, intravenous fluids are necessary for sufficient diastolic filling.
iv. The heart base, right atrium, liver and spleen should be investigated for evidence of masses or tumor infiltrates.

93 i. Check vital signs (circulation, respiration, temperature), neurologic status, and blood glucose.
ii. Surgery-related event; opiate-induced bradycardia; prolonged residual effect of anesthetic agents used (i.e. prolonged sedation, long-duration hypotension); underlying medical problem such as liver disease or shunt; hypoglycemia.
iii. Therapeutic measures depend on findings and may include administration of an anticholinergic if there is a bradycardia, i/v fluids to combat prolonged hypotension, glucose for hypoglycemia, or an opiate antagonist or partial agonist to counter the opiate-related events.

94–96: Questions

94 A two-year-old castrated male Doberman is presented to the emergency service after a fall of 10ft (2m). He has a non-weightbearing lameness of the left front leg (**94**).
i. What is your clinical diagnosis? List possible causes.
ii. What are the next diagnostic steps?
iii. How serious is this problem? What prognosis does each of the potential etiologies suggest and why?

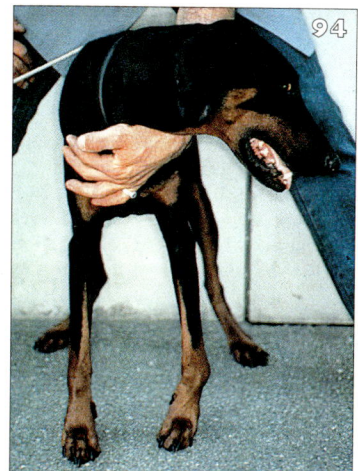

95 A 20 kg male dog is presented for labored breathing 10 hours after falling from the back of a moving truck. Bowel sounds are ausculted in the chest and a diaphragmatic rent is evident on radiographs. The dog is stabilized, anesthetized and intubated and is receiving assisted ventilation. A ventral midline incision from the xyphoid to the pubis is performed with a continuing approach to the thorax via a parasternotomy incision. A ruptured spleen is discovered during abdominal exploration. In addition, the left lateral lobe of the liver and the stomach is displaced into the thorax through a diaphragmatic rent. The prolapsed liver lobe is noted to be swollen and discolored dark purple. The stomach is bruised in appearance and dilated with gas. The lungs appear mildly contused and atalectic.
i. What is the first procedure required?
ii. What are the pros and cons of not amputating this displaced liver lobe?
iii. What are the different methods of partial liver lobectomy?
iv. Describe the procedure for closing the tear in the diaphragm.

96 You are presented with an extremely stressed five-year-old dog. The dog had experienced traumatic shock (middle stage) and multiple trauma with a fractured femur and slight right-sided epistaxis. You need to perform radiography to determine the extent of the hindlimb damage, and to calm the dog and provide analgesia to allow proper clinical evaluation and first aid.
i. What would be your approach to sedation and analgesia in this dog?
ii. Name possible complicating factors that must be considered in these trauma cases if surgical intervention and anesthesia are required.

94–96: Answers

94 i. Varus instability of the left carpal joint. Differential diagnosis at this time includes ulnar collateral ligament injury, avulsion of the ulnar styloid process, intracarpal ligament injury and carpal–metacarpal ligament injury.
ii. Radiographs should be taken under sedation. Craniocaudal and lateral views will detect avulsion fractures. Stressed positions on a craniocaudal view detect widening of one of the joint spaces and help to differentiate the level of injury and the specific ligaments that are involved in this injury.
iii. Ligamentous injuries to the carpal joints are always considered serious. An avulsion of the ulnar styloid process would have a favorable prognosis after stable internal fixation. Lateral carpal injuries are less common than medial injuries and are also less serious than medial collateral ligament injuries. The medial aspects of the carpal joint are under more physiological stress than the lateral aspects because of the valgus position of the carpus of most dogs. Therefore if an attempt is made to repair the lateral ligamentous structures, there is better healing compared with lesions of the medial side of the carpus.

95 i. Control of the splenic hemorrhage by clamping of the affected part or temporarily tying the splenic pedicle with a feeding tube or Penrose drain.
ii. Pros: This liver appears to be ischemic from infarction or trauma. There is a build-up of cytokines in the damaged tissue. Any reperfusion can run the risk of free radical formation and release into the systemic circulation. Necrotic tissue can rupture and cause bleeding during the postoperative period. Also, removal will prevent portal hypertension related to malpositioning of a stretched lobe.
Cons: Increases surgical time and increased risk of intraoperative bleeding.
iii. Parenchymal dissection, electrocoagulation of the smaller vessels, ligation or clipping of the larger vessels.
Parenchymal crushing, with digital pressure of smaller bleeding vessels and ligation of larger vessels.
Stapling with a TA stapler.
iv. The edges of the tear usually do not require debridement. Starting at the most dorsal aspect, the edges are apposed with a non-absorbable monofilament, polygalactin or polydioxanone in a simple continuous, simple interrupted or continuous lock pattern. Circumcostal tears can be sutured to the abdominal wall and around the costal arch.

96 i. Establish an i/v line to start fluid therapy for shock resuscitation.
Supplement oxygen whenever possible before sedation or anesthesia.
If possible, let the dog calm down before any sedation is administered.
Use low-dose opiate–diazepam combination for sedation and analgesia. Refrain from using alpha-blockers due to the risk of significant hypotension.
ii. Hypovolemia, hemorrhage, pneumothorax, ruptured urinary bladder and myocardial and/or lung contusions.

97–99: Questions

97 A 12-year-old, male Golden Retriever presents in severe respiratory distress. Primary survey reveals severe inspiratory stridor that has a loud low-pitched sound associated with it. Mucous membrane color is blue (**97**). Pulmonary auscultation reveals low-pitched, referred upper airway sounds, loudest over the trachea. After an i/v catheter is placed and the dog sedated, oral and pharyngeal examination reveals a swollen, red soft palate and larynx with little mechanical movement of the laryngeal folds. The patient is intubated and receives flow-by oxygen at a fast rate.

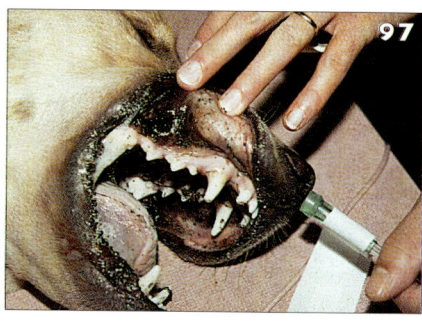

i. What alternatives are there to keeping the patient heavily sedated and intubated?
ii. Describe the procedure for a temporary tracheotomy in an intubated patient versus a catastrophic, awake patient.
iii. List the nursing orders for management of a tracheotomy tube.

98 A previously healthy 3 kg (previously 4.5 kg), castrated male domestic shorthair cat is presented after being trapped within the heating ducts of its house for 3 weeks. The cat was weak and tetraparetic with ventroflexion of the neck, and was emaciated with a persistent skin tent at 10 seconds (**98**). Its eyes were sunken, mucous membranes were pale pink and dry, HR – 180 bpm; RR – 40 bpm; weak peripheral pulses; shallow breathing

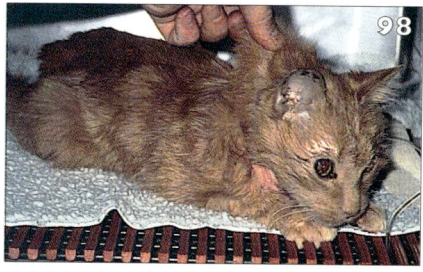

pattern. The urinary bladder was small. Laboratory tests: creatinine – 2.15 mg/dl (190 µmol/l); urea nitrogen – 27.5 mg/dl (11 mmol/l); glucose – 90 mg/dl (5 mmol/l); sodium – 168 mEq/l; potassium – 2.5 mEq/l; albumin – 2.5 g/dl; calculated osmolality – 352 mOsml/l. Venous blood gases: pH – 7.2; HCO_3 – 14 mEq/l; base deficit – 8.0. Urinalysis: SG – 1.060; 1+ ketones.
i. Estimate the degree of dehydration and calculate the fluid volume required to rehydrate this cat.
ii. Select an appropriate type of fluid, electrolyte and vitamin supplement, and justify the choice.
iii. Explain the serum biochemical, blood gas and urine results in this case.
iv. Outline the plan to rehydrate and supplement this cat.

99 With regard to shearing injuries:
i. What would be appropriate wound care?
ii. What type of bandage would you choose?
iii. What is the most important step in the care of this type of wound?
iv. Is surgery necessary? If so, describe.
v. Are antibiotics necessary?

97–99: Answers

97 i. Performing a temporary tracheotomy; placement of a nasotracheal or transtracheal catheter for oxygen supplementation.
ii. Intubated patient: after placing the patient in dorsal recumbency, the ventral cervical region is surgically prepared from the cricothyroid to the distal third of the neck. A local anesthetic is applied. A midline incision is made through the skin over the 4–8th tracheal rings distal to the cricothyroid region. The sternohyoid muscles and fascia are dissected bluntly in a vertical direction, exposing the trachea. A horizontal incision of 50% the diameter of the trachea is made with the scalpel between two rings and sutures placed around the rings distal and proximal to the incision. The sutures are left in a large loop and are used to manipulate the opening for placement of the tracheostomy tube, which is then inserted.
Catastrophic patient: the approach is the same. However, the catastrophic patient may not tolerate sedation or being placed in a dorsally recumbent position because of severe cardiovascular instability. The patient is allowed to remain in a comfortable position with the neck slightly extended. If the patient is in sternal recumbency, the head and neck are extended over the end of a table with the surgeon standing under the head and neck looking up. There may not be enough time to prepare the area surgically.
iii. Nursing care requires daily dressing changes and inspection of the surgical site. The tube should be removed and cleaned, or replaced every 4–6 hours (more often if secretions are increased). The patient should be hyperoxygenated prior to changing the tube. After changing, the airway is suctioned with a clean tube and a small amount of sterile saline should be infused to moisten the airway.

98 i. Estimated 12–15% dehydrated based on the history and physical examination. An animal will lose 0.1–0.3 kg of body weight per day per 1000 kcal energy requirement when deprived of food. Weight lost in excess of this is fluid loss. Assuming 15% dehydration, which is based on current weight, then the fluid deficit is 3 kg $\times$ 0.15 liters = 0.45 liters (450 ml).
ii. Balanced buffered isotonic crystalloid solutions are the fluids of choice. The fluids should be supplemented with KCl (7 mEq/250 ml of fluid). Multiple B vitamins, especially thiamine, should be supplemented and vitamin K given once s/c.
iii. The mild increase in creatinine, urea, sodium and chloride can be explained by deprivation of food and water. The low potassium and albumin is due to starvation and catabolism of body mass. The venous gas levels indicate acidemia (possibly related to ketone production and possibly lactic acid (anion gap = [168 + 2.5] – [14 + 123] = 33). The urine SG suggests good concentration abilities of the kidney; however, it is not known when this urine was produced.
iv. Rehydration must be over 24–48 hours. Total fluids = dehydration deficit + daily maintenance. Potassium should be supplemented up to 0.5 mEq/kg/hour without careful monitoring (1.5 mEq/hour in this cat). Nutrition is provided by tube feeding, beginning with 0.25–1.0 ml/kg/hour glucose/electrolyte solution. If tolerated, this volume can be increased. Nutritional support is then instituted utilizing a dilute liquid diet.

99 i. Open management, debridement, fracture or joint stabilization, allowance for appropriate drainage and antibiotic therapy.
ii. Wet to dry bandages.
iii. Debridement. It should be thorough and done daily at the time of bandage change. Rongeurs may be required to remove non-viable bone fragments. If there is any doubt about the viability of the tissue, it should be left in place until its viability can be determined.
iv. Ligaments may need to be sutured. Screw or wire prosthetic ligaments may be necessary in order to stabilize the affected joint.
v. Antibiotics are usually required. Begin with a broad-spectrum antibiotic and make changes based on culture and sensitivity testing.

100–102: Questions

100 This 18-month-old Boston Terrier was bred 65 days ago (**100**). Temperature is 99°F (37.2°C). The bitch has a clear vaginal discharge and has been having intermittent contractions for 6 hours. The owner is concerned about possible dystocia.
i. Name some breeds in which dystocia is common.
ii. What problems should be ruled out before attempting medical therapy to stimulate uterine contractions?
iii. How can fetal viability best be determined?
iv. What are indications for cesarean section?
v. What anesthetic precautions should be taken for cesarean section?

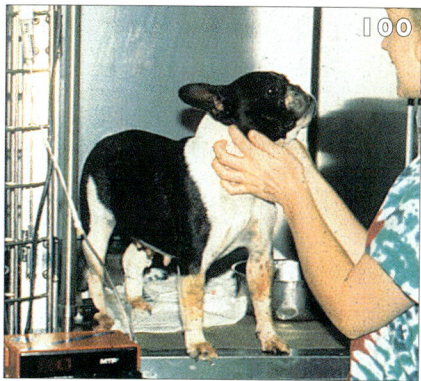

101 This three-year-old, castrated male Golden Retriever presented after being hit by a car (**101**). He is in the middle stage of shock and has sustained a pneumothorax, hemothorax and hemoabdomen. Nasal oxygen was utilized in this patient.
i. What is the pathogenesis for the development of SIRS in this patient?
ii. Why is oxygen supplementation indicated in this patient?
iii. How could the effectiveness of this patient's oxygen therapy be evaluated/monitored?

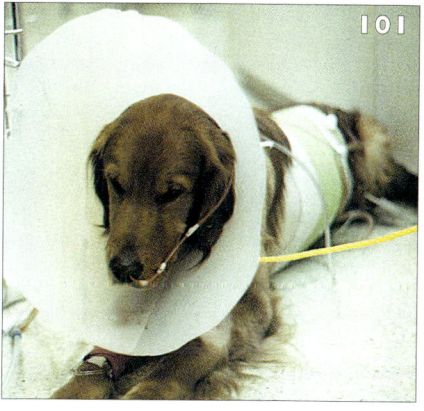

102 For emergency abdominal surgery on a 20 kg mixed-breed dog with signs of an acute abdomen, general anesthesia is achieved with inhalation anesthesia. Patient monitoring consists of ECG and end-tidal CO_2 (concentration in the expiration) recording. You are aware of an acute change in ECG configuration, suggestive of ventricular fibrillation. What three measures, in chronological order, would you immediately take for this patient?

100–102: Answers

100 i. Breeds with large heads and wide shoulders such as Bulldogs, Pugs, Boston Terriers and Scottish Terriers.
ii. Abdominal radiographs and a vaginal examination should be performed. Oxytocin should not be administered if there is evidence of insufficient cervical dilation, vaginal stricture, vaginal mass, uterine torsion or inguinal hernia. Abnormalities of the maternal pelvis, fetal malpositioning and oversized fetuses are also contraindications to oxytocin administration.
iii. Ultrasonography to check for fetal movements and heartbeats is the best method for determining fetal viability. Radiographic signs of fetal death include intrafetal gas patterns, overlapping cranial bones and collapse of the spinal column, but these signs may not be evident until 6–48 hours after fetal death has occurred.
iv. If no response to medical therapy, or if any of the following problems are present: maternal pelvic abnormalities, cephalopelvic disproportion, fetal malpositioning, uterine torsion, uterine inertia and toxicity or illness of the dam.
v. Supplemental oxygen should be provided during induction, as pregnant animals are prone to hypoxia. Also, calculations based on body weight may result in overdose. Because of delayed gastric emptying, pregnant animals are prone to vomiting and aspiration. Systemic antacids and antiemetics can be administered prophylactically to avoid the severe consequences of vomiting and aspiration. Long-acting anesthetic agents which may cause respiratory and cardiovascular depression in the offspring should be avoided. The anesthetic protocol which produces the least fetal depression involves the use of epidural anesthesia and light sedation of the dam. Ultra-short-acting barbiturates will cause respiratory depression and decreased sucking activity. The depression is temporary and these agents can be used for induction at the lowest dose required. Another alternative is propofol (4 mg/kg i/v induction; 0.3–0.5 mg/kg/hour CRI) which has a rapid onset, short duration and smooth recovery when administered as a CRI. Neuroleptanalgesia with diazepam (0.4 mg/kg i/m or i/v) and butorphanol (0.4 mg/kg i/m) can be combined with a local midline block (0.5–1% lidocaine at <10 mg/kg total dosage s/c) or inhalant general anesthesia at the lowest concentration needed. If necessary, neonates can be revived by placing flumazenil (a benzodiazepam antagonist) and naloxone (a narcotic antagonist) on the neonate's tongue. Fluid therapy is important, especially when the uterus is removed from the abdomen, as this results in redistribution of blood volume and possible hypotension.

101 i. The hypovolemic, hemorrhagic shock led to severe sympathetic stimulation and uneven blood flow secondary to vasoconstriction. The hypoxic tissues and local inflammatory response caused by damaged tissue produce toxic mediators of shock such as prostaglandins, thromboxane A2, leukotrienes, kinins, hydrogen ions, proteolytic enzymes, etc. Toxic mediators lead to worsening of perfusion, and a vicious cycle of hypoxic organ death ensues if aggressive resuscitation is not undertaken.
ii. To increase the oxygen delivery to the peripheral tissues due to the supply-dependent oxygen consumption state of SIRS, and because of pulmonary damage and diminished functional pulmonary tissue.
iii. Arterial blood gases, hemoglobin saturation through pulse oximetry.

102
- Check ECG signal for correctness, i.e. differentiate between electrical disturbance and true ventricular fibrillation. Confirm the presence of a cardiovascular collapse with the aid of end-tidal CO_2 and/or peripheral pulse.
- Discontinue administration of all anesthetics and start/continue artificial ventilation with 100% oxygen.
- Take the necessary surgical measures for open chest CPR.

103–105: Questions

103 A six-year-old, castrated male Yorkshire Terrier is presented with a 2-year history of coughing. Today the dog is coughing almost constantly. He has cyanotic mucous membranes and markedly increased inspiratory effort. Radiographs had been taken at a previous visit (**103**).
i. What is the diagnosis?
ii. If radiographs had not confirmed the diagnosis, what additional tests could be performed to diagnose this condition?

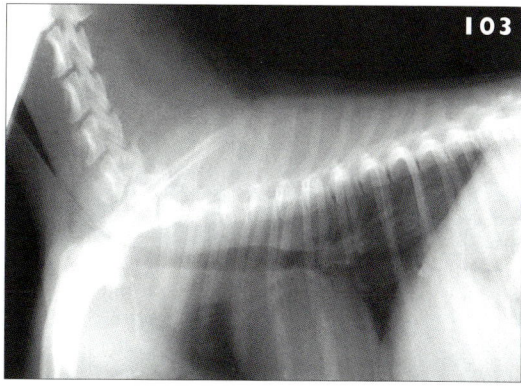

iii. What therapeutic procedures should be instituted immediately?
iv. What medical and surgical options exist for long-term management of this condition?

104 A ten-year-old, male cat was presented for blindness of the right eye (**104**). He is free roaming and returned 2 hours ago reluctant to move. He is lethargic, with ventroflexion of the neck, and is not eating. Physical examination: temperature 103°F (39.4°C), pupil dilated and non-responsive to light in the right eye and normally responsive to light in the left, both direct and consensual. No corneal lacerations were present. The retina is detached in the right eye. The intraocular pressure was normal. The owner reports that the cat has lost weight over the past several weeks and is drinking a lot of water.

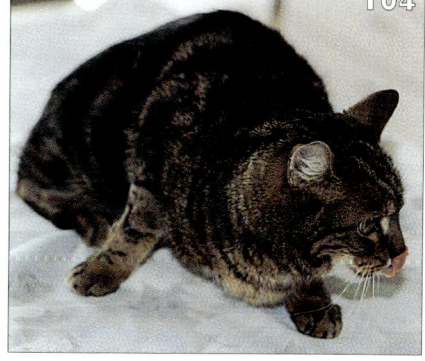

i. What underlying problems are likely to be responsible for the eye problem?
Initial data: PCV – 25%; TS – 8.0 g/dl; creatinine – 5.0 mg/dl (442 µmol/l); Na^+ – 145 mEq/l; K^+ – 1.8 mEq/l; ionized Ca^{++} – 4.8 mg/dl (12 mmol/l); PO_4 – 10 mg/dl (3.23 mmol/l); TCO_2 – 12 mmol/l. Urinalysis: SG – 1.010; protein – 2+; acellular sediment. Systolic blood pressure – 240 mmHg (31.9 kPa) by indirect methods.
ii. What is the likely etiology of the cat's problems?
iii. How would you treat this cat?
iv. What further diagnostics would be required?

105 A nine-week-old puppy is admitted for surgery with signs of diarrhea for 5 days and vomiting for 2 days. Radiographs show an intussusception. What is your general approach to this puppy with regard to supportive measures as well as achieving general anesthesia?

103–105: Answers

103 i. Collapsing trachea.
ii. Radiographs should be taken at full inspiration and full expiration to maximize the possibility that the collapse will be evident on the film. Fluoroscopy, if available, may be more successful at demonstrating an intermittent collapse. Bronchoscopy may allow direct visualization of the collapsing segment, although the trachea may not collapse as dramatically when the dog is under anesthesia. It may be possible to identify weakened tracheal rings and dorsoventral flattening by simple palpation of the cervical region.
iii. Oxygen supplementation. Consider sedation (acepromazine – 0.05 mg/kg i/v or s/c), corticosteroids (prednisolone sodium succinate [2–4 mg/kg i/v] or dexamethasone sodium phosphate [0.2–2.2 mg/kg i/v]) and bronchodilators (aminophylline – 11 mg/kg slow i/v).
iv. Medical management involves the use of bronchodilators (aminophylline or theophylline [10 mg/kg p/o tid] or terbutaline [1.25–5.0 mg/dog p/o bid–tid]), cough suppressants (butorphanol [0.5 mg/kg p/o bid–qid], hydrocodone [0.25 mg/kg p/o bid–tid], dextromethorphan [2.2 mg/kg p/o bid–tid]) and anti-inflammatory agents (prednisone – 0.25–0.5 mg/kg p/o bid). A search for a bacterial component of bronchitis is warranted.
There are several surgical options. These include plication of the dorsal tracheal membrane, tracheal ring resection, placement of internal stents or external prosthetic rings, or spiral prosthesis. Careful examination for laryngeal paralysis is indicated before surgical correction.

104 i. Hypertension, infiltrative diseases such as fungal disease, lymphosarcoma, FIP.
ii. Chronic renal disease with hypokalemic myopathy and hypertension. The renal pathology can be due to interstitial fibrosis, infiltrative disease in the kidneys or hyperthyroidism.
iii. I/v fluids and diuresis, potassium supplementation, amlodipine.
iv. Abdominal radiographs, abdominal ultrasound, T3, T4, FeLV, FIV, kidney aspirate, echocardiography.

105
- Start i/v fluid therapy with crystalloids and colloids. Check and correct electrolyte and acid–base imbalances (particularly hypokalemia, hypomagnesemia, hypophosphatemia and metabolic acidosis). Check off the following dos and do nots:
- Pre-oxygenate before induction.
- Premedicate with low dose atrophine or glycopyrrolate.
- Ensure adquate analgesia pre-, intra- and postoperatively.
- Beware of cardiovascular depressant anesthetics; preferably use a narcotic–tranquilizer combination (such as fentanyl–droperidol or oxymorphone–diazepam) which will allow a lower concentration of isoflurane instead of inducing with a vasodilating sedative such as barbiturates or propofol. Use anesthetics which are not metabolized by the liver and which can be antagonized. Nitrous oxide is contraindicated as an adjuctive inhalation gas in this dog with bowel surgery.

106–108: Questions

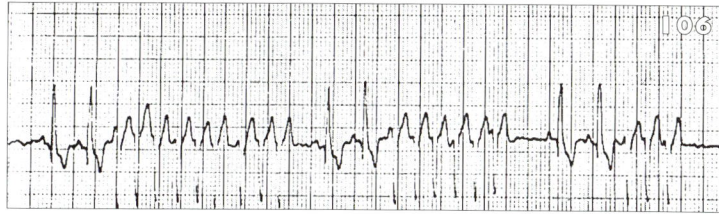

106 A three-year-old, spayed female Great Dane presented recumbent with abdominal distension. She received 4 liters of lactated Ringer's solution i/v and remained recumbent with pale mucous membranes. She was decompressed with an orogastric tube. On auscultation, HR is rapid and pulses are barely palpable.
i. What is the ECG diagnosis (**106**; speed 25 mm/sec)?
ii. What interventions are necessary at this time?
iii. What are possible adverse reactions to drug treatment, and how should they be treated?
iv. What are possible causes of this dog's new problem, and what diagnostics would be indicated?

107 A four-year-old Yorkshire Terrier presented with a relatively sudden onset unilateral (left) painful eye. There were no other problems but the owners considered that the dog had experienced some discomfort during the previous 2 days. On the morning of the consultation there had been marked blepharospasm and excessive lacrimation. Examination revealed conjunctival and episcleral congestion and a diffuse mild corneal edema (**107**). There was a faint misty appearance to the anterior chamber and the pupil was constricted.
i. Describe the pathology seen in the eye.
ii. What is your diagnosis?
iii. What would you expect tonometry to reveal?
iv. What treatment would you prescribe?

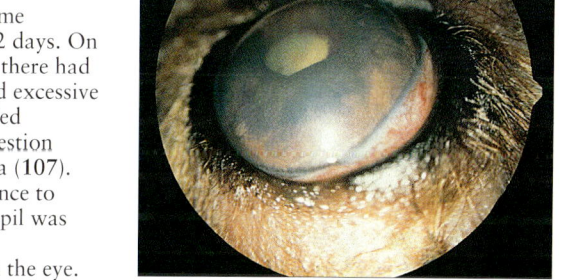

108 An owner is 90 minutes away from your facility and calls for advice about his dog that ran through a plate glass window and is actively bleeding from the right forelimb.
i. What are your recommendations concerning first aid?
ii. What are your recommendations concerning transport?

106–108: Answers

106 i. Paroxysmal ventricular tachycardia at a ventricular rate of 300 bpm.
ii. A slow intravenous bolus of lidocaine 2% (2–4 mg/kg) is given. This dose can be repeated if there is poor or no response. Once converted to sinus rhythm, an i/v continuous lidocaine infusion (50–75 µg/kg/minute) is given. Alternatively, a slow i/v procainamide bolus is given and a continuous infusion (11–40 µg/kg/minute) started after conversion. Bretyllium can be given i/v, allowing 20 minutes for the full effect. If, however, conversion to sinus rhythm is unsuccessful by medical intervention, electrical defibrillation (can start with 100 J) is an option as this can precede sustained ventricular tachycardia and fibrillation.
iii. The risk of profound hypotension associated with too rapid infusion. Also, gastrointestinal side-effects may occur but are transient and eliminated at lower dosages. With lidocaine, increased dosage may cause ataxia or seizures which can be treated with i/v diazepam and discontinuation of the drug.
iv. Causes include hypoxia, acid–base or electrolyte disturbances and myocardial irritability secondary to toxemia. Also, Great Danes are predisposed to dilated cardiomyopathy which may go undetected until a serious illness. Obtaining an arterial blood gas and eletrolytes (to include K^+ and Mg^{++}) and appropriate treatment to correct these abnormalities should precede surgical gastric repositioning. Chest radiographs and an echocardiogram should be included in the pretoperative monitoring.

107 i. The anterior chamber contains inflammatory product (flare) and the iris sphincter muscle is in spasm.
ii. Acute uveitis of unknown aetiology.
iii. A low intraocular pressure.
iv. Topical and systemic anti-inflammatory drugs and a topical cycloplegic agent to break the ciliary spasm and reduce the discomfort are needed. Atropine is both a mydriatic and a cycloplegic, the mydriasis again helping to relieve the discomfort but reducing the chances of posterior synechiae formation.

108 i. Restraint of the animal is required and a muzzle made of long pieces of cloth may be necessary. Hemostasis is first accomplished by direct pressure applied over the wound. If the blood is dark and oozing (venous), elevating the leg and applying a small compression bandage can reduce bleeding. If the blood is red and pumping (arterial), a snug compression bandage is necessary. When the bandage becomes blood soaked, additional material is placed over the original bandage. If compression bandages do not prevent active bleeding, a tourniquet is placed above the bleeding site and loosened every 10 minutes and then retightened.
ii. Transport must be immediate. The dog must be kept quiet.

109 & 110: Questions

109 Enteral feeding of the critically ill patient has been shown to be useful in decreasing morbidity and mortality.
i. Name five reasons why this should be so.
   Your patient requires abdominal surgery. You decide a feeding tube should be placed.
ii. Briefly describe how an esophagostomy tube is placed.
iii. How is a jejunostomy tube placed? Give five indications for placing a jejunostomy tube.
iv. Name three potential complications of transabdominal feeding tubes.

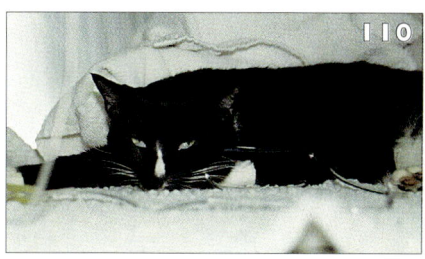

110 A seven-year-old spayed female domestic shorthair cat (6 kg) is presented with a history of polyuria/polydipsia for several days' duration, inappropriate urination and vomiting of 1 day's duration. The patient presents in lateral recumbency with depressed mentation, but is responsive to pain. HR – 160 bpm; RR – 60 bpm; rectal temperature – 97°F (36.1°C); mucous membranes are gray; CRT – 4 seconds. The femoral pulses are weak and there are no palpable dorsal pedal pulses. The cat is estimated as 8% dehydrated. Initial data base reveals: PCV – 45%; TS – 8.0 g/dl; BUN labstick – 50–80 mg/dl; glucose labstick >400 mg/dl (>22.4 mmol/l).
i. Select the appropriate initial therapeutic procedure for this cat:
a. Apply warm water bottles to raise the body temperature.
b. Give 5 units regular insulin s/c.
c. Give supplemental oxygen by oxygen cage.
d. Give i/v fluids until perfusion has improved.
e. Administer dopamine (10 µg/kg/minute).
   Additional blood work finds: Na^+ – 156 mEq/l; K^+ – 3.05 mEq/l; chloride – 116 mEq/l; Ca^{++} (ionized) – 3.67 mg/dl (0.92 mmol/l); arterial blood gas: pH – 7.20, HCO_3 – 17 mEq/l, $PaCO_2$ – 34 mmHg (4.5 kPa); anion gap – 30 mEq/l; creatinine = 2.28 mg/dl (201.6 µmol/l) (normal 0.80–2.40 mg/dl [70.7–212.2 µmol/l]). Urinalysis: SG – 1.026; ketones negative; glucose – 2000+; occasional epithelial cell on sediment.
ii. Select the most appropriate rehydration plan:
a. 0.9% saline replacing 240 ml fluid deficit over 12 hours.
b. 0.45% saline replacing 480 ml fluid deficit over 8 hours.
c. Lactated Ringer's solution replacing 480 ml fluid deficit over 12 hours
d. Lactated Ringer's solution replacing 240 ml deficit over 8 hours.
iii. What are the mechanisms for the hypokalemia on presentation?
iv. Because the urine tested negative on a dipstick for ketones, what other indicator does this cat have that there could be ketones present?
v. What would be the most appropriate insulin therapy for this cat?
vi. What mechanism is responsible for the hyponatremia, sometimes called pseudohyponatremia, often seen on presentation with diabetes ketoacidosis?
vii. It is safe to rehydrate the animal quickly because the brain forms idiogenic osmoles which will maintain normal hydration of the brain in spite of abrupt serum osmolality changes. True or false?

109 & 110: Answers

109 i. Enteral nutrition helps maintain the gut barrier, thus decreasing bacterial translocation. The hypermetabolic response has been shown to be decreased. Immunologic function is maintained and wound healing is improved.
ii. Curved hemostats are inserted past the pharynx into the proximal esophagus. The tips of the hemostats are pushed upward to make an obvious bulge. A skin incision is made over the tips and the tips are forced through the esophagus, s/c and skin. The tip of the tube is grasped, pulled into the esophagus and out through the mouth. The tube is then redirected down the esophagus until the tip rests in the caudal thoracic esophagus. The tube is secured by suturing to the skin and deep fascia of the atlas.
iii. A 3.5–8 French gauge feeding tube is placed through a stab incision in the left lateral abdominal wall at the level of the proximal jejunum. A purse-string suture of 4-0 monofilament suture is placed in the antimesenteric border of the proximal jejunum. A stab incision is made inside the purse-string and the tube fed aborally 10–12 cm into the jejunum. The purse-string is tightened and a single suture placed inside the ostomy and tied to the tube to prevent migration. A continuous circumferential 'to-and-fro' suture is placed between the jejunum and the abdominal wall and tightened so that the jejunum is anchored against the abdominal wall. Omentum is then sutured around the ostomy site. The tube is anchored by suturing the tube to the skin and fascia.
  Indications include pancreatitis; upper GI tract surgery (cholangiohepatic, gastric, duodenal); gastroparesis; risk for aspiration postoperatively due to neurologic status; multiple surgeries required where gastric feedings would need to be withheld for several days or more.
iv. The ostomy site may break down, causing leakage of abdominal contents or feedings into the fascia and leading to a necrotizing fasciitis; the tube may become dislodged, leading to administration of feedings intraperitoneally; the gastric or intestinal wall may necrose around the tube if sutures are inappropriately placed.

110 i. d.
ii. c.
iii. Potassium is lost due to the osmotic diuresis produced by hyperglycemia. Sodium and potassium salts of the ketoacids are formed and these are excreted by the kidney. The acidosis causes movement of K^+ from the cell into the serum.
iv. Anion gap.
v. It has been shown that an i/v CRI of regular insulin, or low dose regular insulin given hourly i/m, will slowly decrease the glucose and serum osmolality. Once the blood glucose has become normal and the animal is hydrated and eating, s/c insulin can be given.
vi. A flux of fluid from intracellular to extracellular spaces occurs due to the hyperosmolality due to the hyperglycemia. This can have a dilutional effect on the serum sodium.
vii. False.

111 & 112: Questions

111 A five-year-old mixed-breed dog presents in acute cardiorespiratory arrest. The owner directs you to initiate resuscitative efforts.
i. Define basic and advanced life support.
ii. List in order of priority your procedures for basic life support.
iii. List in order of priority your procedures for advanced life support.
iv. What significance does the term cardiopulmonary cerebral resuscitation (CPCR) have in describing your resuscitative efforts?
v. Chest compression during closed chest CPCR promotes blood flow by what two methods?
vi. List advantages and disadvantages of closed and open chest CPCR.
vii. Ventilations and chest compressions are not producing adequate perfusion for resuscitative efforts. What other technique can be employed if the owner does not want open chest CPCR?
viii. The dog presented without a catheter. Give four routes for rapid administration of epinephrine, lidocaine and atropine during CPCR that do not require direct venous access. How are the drugs dosed for these routes?
ix. Name the five most common arrhythmias associated with the no-flow state of cardiopulmonary arrest.
x. Match the following drugs with their intended action in CPCR:

Epinephrine	**Parasympatholytic activity**
Atropine	**Correct myocardial acidosis**
Lidocaine	**Convert fine to coarse fibrillation**
Sodium bicarbonate	**Support heart and blood pressure post CPR**
Dopamine	**Stop re-entry phenomonon**

112 A three-year-old, spayed female mixed-breed dog presents with severe intravascular hemolysis and vomiting. An abdominal radiograph reveals a circular radiopaque metallic density in the stomach (**112**).
i. What is the most likely cause for the hemolytic crisis based on the limited information given?
ii. What are the major systems affected by this intoxication?
iii. What is/are specific treatments for this intoxication?

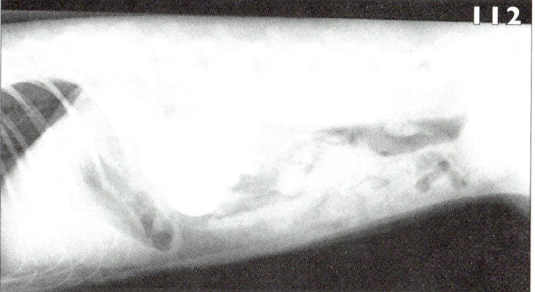

111 & 112: Answers

111 i. Basic life support is airway, breathing and closed chest compressions to promote circulation. Advanced life support includes ECG interpretation, drug administration, defibrillation and open chest cardiac massage.
ii. Check the dog for respirations, pulses and heart beat; examine the back of the throat for obstruction; obtain an airway and begin ventilation (mouth to nose if no equipment is available) and intubation and positive pressure ventilation with 100% oxygen if available. Give 3–4 strong breaths to begin with and reassess pulses and heart beat. If absent, begin closed chest compressions at 60–100 compressions per minute.
iii. Attach an ECG and assess the rate and rhythm; administer appropriate drugs and/or defibrillation; reassess adequacy of basic life support procedures; determine and perform open chest cardiac massage if considered necessary; drugs and defibrillation as necessary; volume expansion as necessary; support of BP if CPCR successful; methods to lower intracranial pressure if successful; surgical repair of problems leading to or resulting from CPR if successful.
iv. The cardiovascular and pulmonary systems and the brain must be resuscitated. It is futile to re-establish blood flow and respirations if the brain is permanently and severely damaged. The term reminds the resuscitators that careful attention must be given to re-establishing brain function, protecting the brain from injury and hypoxia, and making conditions post resuscitation the best for decreasing intracranial pressure and promoting cerebral perfusion pressures.
v. Direct cardiac compression and the thoracic pump.
vi. Closed: advantages include no surgical time, immediate initiation, lower cost; disadvantages are that it may not provide sufficient perfusion, does not allow examination of the thoracic cavity, larger sized dogs do not get the benefit of direct cardiac massage. Open: advantages include direct examination of the intrathoracic structures, immediate vascular access, ability to estimate intravascular volume, ability to cross-clamp aorta, visual and palpable assessment of cardiac contractility, better ability to increase perfusion to the head and heart; disadvantages are that it requires surgical skills for closure if successful, there is potential for infection if done outside of OR, increased costs.
vii. Abdominal counterpressure.
viii. Intratracheal – twice the usual CPCR dosage; sublingual – twice the usual CPCR dosage; intracardiac – normal CPCR dosage; intraosseous – normal CPCR dosage.
ix. Asystole; ventricular fibrillation; pulseless idioventricular rhythm; electrical/mechanical dissociation; ventricular flutter.
x.

Epinephrine	Convert fine to coarse fibrillation
Atropine	Parasympatholytic activity
Lidocaine	Stop re-entry phenomenon
Sodium bicarbonate	Correct myocardial acidosis
Dopamine	Support heart and blood pressure post CPCR

112 i. Zinc-induced hemolysis secondary to ingestion of zinc-containing metallic objects such as US pennies minted before 1983 or certain transport cage nuts.
ii. RBCs, and the kidney and GI system.
iii. Eliminate the source of zinc by removal of the metallic object and then supportive care, particularly transfusions with packed RBCs.

113–115: Questions

113 Two dogs present to your hospital at the same time. One has an open fracture of the left femur with HR – 140 bpm; temperature – 101.9°F (38.8°C); RR – 40 bpm; CRT – 1 second; mucous membranes – pink. The other dog is vomiting with HR – 180 bpm; temperature – 101.8°F (38.8°C); RR – 40 bpm; CRT – 3 seconds; mucous membranes – gray.
i. After triage assessment, how would you prioritize these two dogs?
ii. What is your immediate management of the most critical patient?
iii. What first aid would you provide to the waiting animal?

114 A dog presents to your hospital in shock. It had attempted to jump out of a boat and had landed on the edge of a dock. A diagnosis of severe intra-abdominal hemorrhage is made and the dog is taken to surgery for an exploratory laparotomy (**114**). You suspect liver trauma.
i. What is the significance of the portal triad with reference to control of hemorrhage?
ii. What is the name for the maneuver that occludes the portal triad?

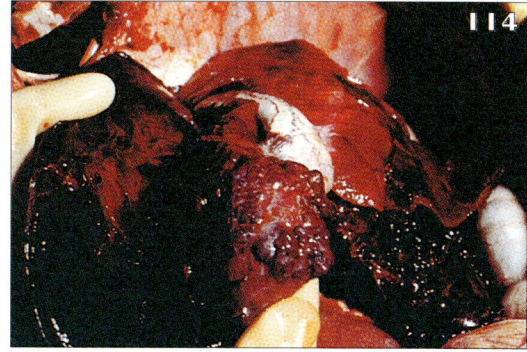

iii. Name six intraoperative methods of controlling hemorrhage to the liver.
iv. Attempts at controlling the hemorrhage from multiple liver fractures were not completely successful and there is still generalized oozing. What is the next step?
v. Major bleeding in the liver can arise from what five major areas?

115 A four-year-old, entire male Miniature Pinscher is presented 1 hour after a fight with a German Shepherd Dog. On physical examination he has a HR of 160 bpm and weak femoral pulses. Two lacerations are noted on the right side of the chest wall, two small puncture wounds on both sides of the chest wall and two small puncture wounds on both sides of the abdomen. The right forelimb has a large open wound with fracture of the radius and ulna.
i. What are your immediate concerns?
ii. What is your diagnostic and treatment plan?
iii. How would you treat the wounds?
iv. How would you monitor the dog, and what complications are anticipated?

113–115: Answers

113 i. The vomiting dog is in the early decompensatory stage of shock and has priority.
ii. Oxygen, i/v catheter, draw pretreatment blood and urine, administer crystalloids (possibly colloids), monitor ECG and BP.
iii. The open fracture is covered with moist sterile gauze and placed in a support wrap. Analgesics are administered if the cardiovascular system is stable. The dog is observed closely during the wait because of the history of trauma.

114 i. Occlusion of the portal triad is used to control hemorrhage to the liver.
ii. The Pringle maneuver.
iii. Direct pressure, packing, suturing, omental packing, hemostatic agents and superglue.
iv. The abdomen should be packed with towels or laparotomy pads, closed temporarily and re-explored in 24–72 hours. Blood/plasma products should be given as needed to replace clotting factors.
v. The portal vein, hepatic artery, hepatic vein, retrohepatic vena cava and deep parenchyma. Major bleeding carries a guarded prognosis due to the difficulty in controlling hemorrhage definitively, the need for multiple transfusions and the high incidence of DIC postoperatively.

115 i. The dog shows signs of middle stage (early decompensatory) shock. The shock and the chest injury could lead to tissue hypoxia. The shearing forces that occur when a small dog is picked up and swung by a larger dog can cause head, neck, spine and other injuries that may not be obvious. The bite wounds are only the 'tip of the iceberg' – with the surface not reflecting the depth and extent of muscle and fascial injuries. Bite wounds are a source of infection, with bacteria injected deep into the tissues. Cellulitis and sepsis can occur from the tissue damage and necrosis. Penetration into the chest and abdomen are possible with the dog suddenly developing a sucking chest wound or peritonitis from bowel rupture.
ii. The first choice of treatment is volume expansion with crystalloids such as lactated Ringer's solution and colloids such as hetastarch. Oxygen is given by flow-by or hood techniques. Analgesic are administered. Antibiotics effective against Gram-positive and Gram-negative aerobic and anaerobic bacteria are given i/v. Thoracocentesis may be required. Serial monitoring of PVC, TS, HR, RR, glucose, BP and breathing pattern is necessary. Thoracic radiographs, once the animal is stabilized, will better define pleural space, pulmonary and thoracic wall injury. An ECG and neurologic examination will determine cardiac and neurologic status.
iii. Once the animal is stabilized the wounds should be explored and damaged and dead tissue debrided. General anesthesia is required, providing adequate BP support during induction and maintenance. The surgeon must be prepared to enter the chest and abdomen at any time during exploration. The bite wounds should be laid open, thoroughly cleaned and any discolored or infected muscles, fat or tissues excised. A suction drain is placed and protected and stabilized with bandage material. The open fracture wound should be thoroughly explored and flushed. Surgical stabilization will be based on radiographic evaluation of the fracture site. Immediate stabilization is optional.
iv. If there is no penetration into body cavities, the dog should be monitored for signs of shock, cardiac dysfunction, tissue oxygenation, RR and respiratory effort. Systemic infection is possible. Extensive wounds will cause loss of fluid and protein. The dog should be monitored for onset of SIRS. Monitoring should include: PCV/TS, albumin, coagulation, temperature, HR, CRT, mucous membrane color, RR and pattern, CVP, BP, saturation of oxygen, electrolytes and glucose.

116–118: Questions

116 You are presented with a three-year-old, castrated male cat (6 kg) with a 2-day history of vomiting, and straining in the litter pan (**116**). On presentation the cat has a hard non-expressable bladder with an extended penis, and he appears to be 8% dehydrated. Gum color is pink; HR – 200 bpm; CRT – 2 seconds.
i. Comment on the use of hypertonic saline in this patient.
ii. What is your plan for fluid resuscitation and maintenance?

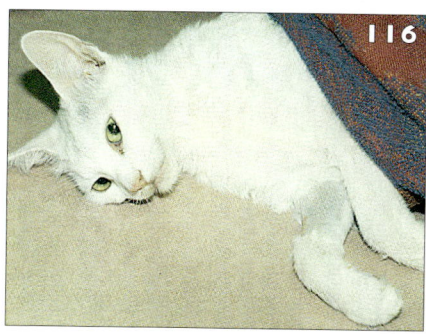

117 Your triage nurse alerts you that a three-year-old, male Coonhound (40 kg) with a few hours' history of non-productive retching and pacing has entered the hospital (**117a**). Primary survey reveals poor perfusion, rapid and irregular heart rate, and a tympanic, distended cranial abdomen. A lateral radiograph reveals gastric dilatation and volvulus.
i. What are the pros and cons of the following surgical procedures for preventing gastric volvulus from recurring: circumcostal gastropexy; antral incisional gastropexy; tube gastropexy; midline abdominal closure gastropexy?
ii. What vessels are most commonly torn during a gastric dilatation/volvulus episode, and where are these located?
iii. What surgical findings would indicate that a splenectomy is required?

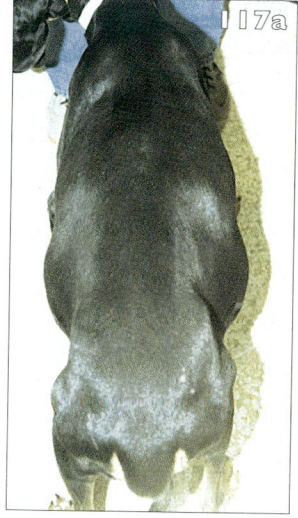

118 This two-year-old dog presented for acute collapse (**118**). On primary survey you note that his gum color is white and he has rapid, shallow breathing. HR is 200 bpm and the femoral pulses are not palpable. You cannot hear lung sounds on pulmonary auscultation. Initial data base: PCV – 12%; TS – 2.0 g/dl. The owner reports that the dog had access to an anticoagulant rodenticide several days ago.
i. What are the pathophysiologic causes of tissue hypoxia in this patient?
ii. What are the pathophysiologic results of cellular hypoxia?
iii. What therapeutic actions would you perform to restore cellular metabolism?

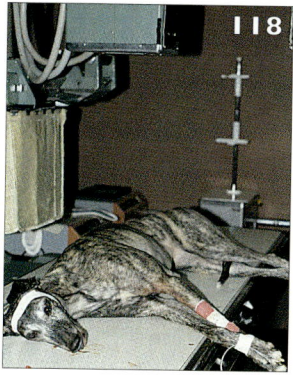

116–118: Answers

116 i. I/v hypertonic saline has the immediate effect of pulling in water from the interstitial space. However, interstitial fluid content is low in a dehydrated patient. Therefore, it is not recommended for use in this patient as it would dehydrate him further.
ii. I/v isotonic crystalloids need to be given, not only to diurese but also to correct dehydration. In this case, after unobstructing the cat, the fluid rate should be 6 kg × 0.08 = 0.420 liters/6 hours = 80 ml/hour, plus 2 ml/kg/hour maintenance fluid (100 ml/hour + 10 ml/hour diuresis = 110 ml/hour for the first 6 hours). These cats will typically develop a postobstructive diuresis due to back pressure on the renal tubules from the bladder. Calculating their fluid requirements is sometimes difficult without measuring urine output. One could add the maintenance rate (2 ml/kg/hour) to the hourly urine output, adding any replacement fluids for dehydration. This may seem like a large amount of fluid, but it is required. Pulmonary auscultation should occur as part of the regular nursing orders to monitor for fluid overload.

117 i. Circumcostal gastropexy. Pros: most reliable adhesions obtained. Cons: time-consuming preparation; potential for rib fractures; potential for entering pleural space and causing pneumothorax.

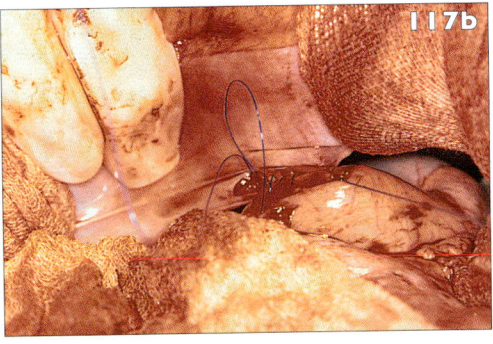

Antral incisional gastropexy (**117b**). Pros: rapid technique with less technical difficulty. Cons: none.
Tube gastropexy. Pros: ability for postoperative decompression and feeding control. Cons: requires time for fistula formation before tube can be removed; requires exposure of the gastric lumen.
Midline abdominal closure gastropexy. Pros: rapid technique. Cons: makes a reapproach to the cranial abdomen very difficult.
ii. Short gastric arteries and left epiploic artery along the greater curvature of the fundus.
iii. Dark/black areas suggesting an infarction/ischemia; lack of palpable pulses in the splenic hilus suggesting arterial thrombosis; disseminated masses that may be neoplastic; bleeding mass; uncontrollable hemorrhage of the spleen.

118 i. There is evidence of poor ventilation, hypovolemia and a decreased red cell mass.
ii. When cells are deprived of oxygen, the cellular pump mechanisms dysfunction, resulting in an accumulation of sodium, calcium and water in the cell. Cellular swelling causes disruption of the cell membrane followed by release of arachidonic acid and production of leukotrienes and prostaglandins. Toxic oxygen radicals are also produced during cellular hypoxia.
iii. Firstly, respiratory support is required in the form of oxygen supplementation and possible thoracocentesis if pleural air or effusion is suspected. Red cell replacement is required in the form of a whole blood transfusion. Added fluid support in the form of isotonic crystalloids is also recommended to improve perfusion. Treatment for the underlying cause is paramount for preventing further hemorrhage.

119–121: Questions

119 This two-year-old, FeLV-positive, entire male cat presented for anorexia and lethargy. Physical examination revealed: pale mucous membranes; RR – 80 bpm; HR – 240 bpm. PCV – 7%; TS – 8.0 g/dl.
i. Which infectious disease would be likely to be causing the anemia in this FeLV-positive cat?
ii. Would you expect the anemia to be regenerative or non-regenerative?
iii. Describe your protocol for transfusing this cat.

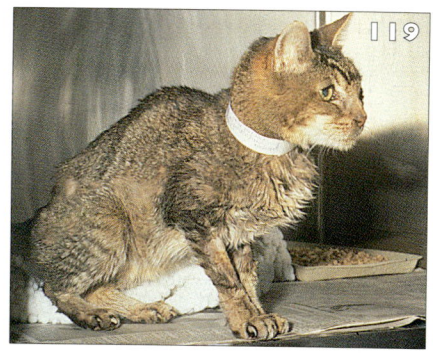

120 A five-year-old, female Cocker Spaniel-cross was tied to the trailer hitch of the family automobile. The family forgot she was there and drove away, dragging her almost 1/4 mile. She presented ambulatory and in stable condition but was extremely painful. Not only did she have the wounds pictured (**120**), but she had similar wounds on her left side inguinally, and on her left forelimb as well.
i. One of the following should **NOT** be done for initial management of her

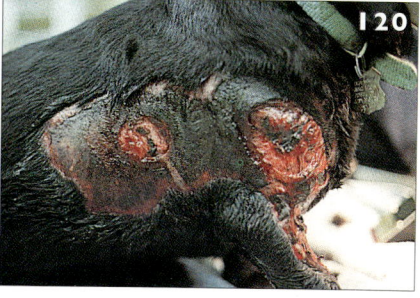

wounds: general anesthesia; liberal hair removal around the wounds; copious lavage with sterile saline or other physiologic solution; surgical debridement; thorough cleansing of wounds and skin with chlorhexidine; wet to dry dressings.
ii. How long will these wounds take to heal? Days, weeks, months or will likely never heal completely?
iii. What dressings would you recommend once healthy granulation tissue has formed?
iv. List tension relieving techniques that will aid in closure of this wound should delayed closure be chosen as the appropriate treatment.
v. List goals of wound debridement.

121 A six-year-old, male German Shepherd Dog-cross is depressed and weak on presentation and has a rapid RR. Mucous membranes are pale with a prolonged CRT, femoral pulses are weak, jugular veins are distended with pulsation, and hepatosplenomegaly is apparent. A loud murmur is present on the right and a split S_2 is auscultated. During the examination the dog urinates a port wine coloured urine.
i. What is your tentative diagnosis?
ii. Prior to echocardiography, what diagnostics could provide valuable information?
iii. What supportive treatment would you initiate?

119–121: Answers

119 i. *Haemobartonella felis* is a common cause of anemia in FeLV positive cats.
ii. Typically, FeLV is associated with macrocytosis; however, cats with *H. felis* infection may be normocytic (MVC – 60–70 fl) and non-regenerative.
iii. Generally, whole blood is administered to cats requiring RBC transfusion. Whole blood can be withdrawn from a donor cat by sedating the donor with ketamine (2–4 mg/kg i/v). Typically, approximately 50–60 ml of blood can be withdrawn from the donor cat into a syringe containing 9 ml of acid citrate dextrose (7 ml of blood/ml of acid citrate dextrose). The volume and rate of blood administered varies with the patient's clinical signs and laboratory data. In general, 2 ml/kg of whole blood will increase the patient's PCV by 1%. The transfusion rate for whole blood should be 5 mg/kg during a 4-hour period or, if the patient is hypovolemic, 5 ml/kg/hour. The first 10 ml should be given slowly over a 15 minute period to observe for adverse reactions. Blood should always be administered through an appropriate filter and administration set designed to retain blood clots and other debris.

120 i. Chlorhexidine and povidone–iodine surgical scrub solution should never be allowed in contact with the exposed or damaged tissues.
ii. Months. Bandage changes may be 1–2 times per day initially, and then every 2–3 days after the first week.
iii. Non-adherent dressings are recommended because they do not disturb developing granulation tissue (capillary loops and collagen).
iv. Tension relieving techniques include undermining, vertical mattress sutures, stented sutures, relaxing incisions, bipedicle flaps or V-Y or Z plasty.
v. Remove all devitalized or necrotic tissue; remove all foreign bodies and debris; provide careful hemostasis; irrigate the wound copiously; preserve vital structures.

121 i. Heartworm caval syndrome. Hemoglobinuria is pathognomonic.
ii.
• *Laboratory tests*: microfilaremia (85%); hemoglobinemia, regenerative anemia, schistocytes and spherocytes due to RBC fragility and hemolysis; possible leukocytosis with neutrophilia, eosinophilia, left shift; increased liver enzymes (thrombosis and necrosis) and possibly increased renal enzymes (tubular necrosis); also hypoalbuminemia, hyperglobulinemia and hyperbilirubinemia. Metabolic acidosis and coagulation abnormalities (if DIC) may also be present.
• *ECG*: include atrial or ventricular premature complexes.
• *Chest radiographs*: cardiomegaly, main pulmonary artery enlargement, pulmonary artery tortuosity.
iii. Fluid therapy is important to improve cardiac output and tissue perfusion, correct metabolic acidosis, prevent DIC and prevent ongoing renal tubular necrosis from hemoglobinuria. CVP should be monitored closely and should not be permitted to exceed 10 cmH$_2$O (0.98 kPa). Catheter placement should be left jugular and should not extend to the cranial vena cava. Aspirin to prevent thromboembolism and broad-spectrum antibiotics are recommended. Heparin should be substituted for aspirin if DIC is suspected. Removal of worms from the vena cava is often required.

122 & 123: Questions

122 A nine-year-old, female mixed-breed dog was diagnosed as having endometritis and was treated with gentamicin (4 mg/kg i/m every 8 hours). The dog was presented for a second opinion since it was oliguric, dehydrated, anorexic and vomiting. Blood tests revealed: PCV – 56%; TS – 8.0 g/dl; creatinine – 10 mg/dl (884 µmol/l); BUN – 250 mg/dl; phosphorus – 4.0 mg/dl; blood glucose – 80 mg/dl (4.48 mmol/l); Na^+ – 158 mEq/l; K^+ –

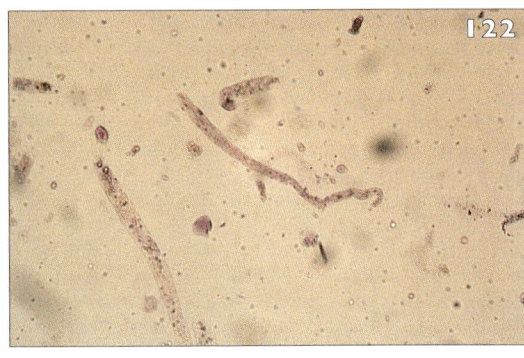

4.0 mEq/l; albumin – 2.5 g/dl. Urinalysis revealed: SG – 1.010; proteinuria – 1+; glucose – 1+; granular casts/hpf – 0–5 (**122**).
i. What is your assessment of the renal status?
ii. What is your tentative diagnosis?
iii. What prognosis do you give the owners?
iv. What is your therapeutic approach ?

123 A patient presents with evidence of a gunshot wound to the cranial abdomen. No exit wound is seen. As the patient is being fluid resuscitated, progressive abdominal distension is noted and despite fluids, the patient's femoral pulses are still not palpable. Suspecting severe abdominal hemorrhage, abdominal counterpressure is placed (**123**).
i. What is abdominal counterpressure?

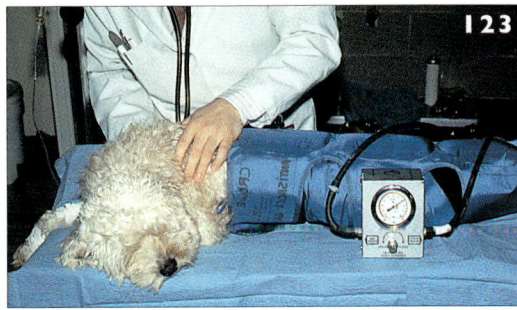

ii. What is the principle behind abdominal counterpressure?
iii. If a commercial pneumatic antishock garment is not available, what common materials can be used?
iv. How tight should the garment be placed, and how can this be assessed?
v. What may happen if it is placed too tightly?
vi. When placing abdominal counterpressure, what parts of the body should be included and why?

External counterpressure is applied. The patient's respiratory effort starts to become labored and the dog starts to appear anxious.
vii. What are the most likely causes of the anxiety?
viii. What are the most likely causes of the increase in respiratory effort?
ix. What are the four most likely internal injuries present if an increase in respiratory effort is noted?
x. What should be done to assist the patient's with counterpressure and an increase in respiratory effort?
xi. When should abdominal counterpressure be avoided?

122 & 123: Answers

122 i. The severe azotemia with a fixed SG is indicative of primary renal failure. There is most likely a prerenal component with the dehydration; however, the parameters are too elevated to be prerenal alone. The normal PCV and phosphorus suggest that the renal injury is acute rather than chronic. The glycosuria in the face of normal blood glucose and a high number of granular casts are compatible with renal tubular necrosis, particularly proximal tubular damage. The high dose of gentamicin in the face of dehydration is a likely etiology.
ii. Gentamicin-induced acute tubular necrosis.
iii. Guarded to poor.
iv. If a gentamicin overdose has been given, immediate peritoneal dialysis can be effective in removing the excess gentamicin from the blood stream. However, once renal tubular damage has occurred, supportive care to allow tubular regeneration is the mainstay of therapy. I/v crystalloids are given to replace perfusion and hydration and promote diuresis. Monitoring of CVP, BP and urine output are important. Should oliguria occur, early infusion of mannitol (0.1 g/kg i/v) can be given. If it is successful at re-establishing urine output, a 10% mannitol drip is used. If it is unsuccessful, then furosemide (1 mg/kg i/v by CRI for 4 hours) combined with dopamine (1–3 µg/kg/minute CRI) are administered. Blood gases are monitored for metabolic acidosis and the acidosis treated if it persists after rehydration. Vomiting should be controlled and the consequences of uremia, such as gastric ulceration, malnutrition, vasculitis and bleeding disorders, treated.

123 i. The placement of external pressure over the abdomen.
ii. Pressure is placed on vessels indirectly, causing a decrease in the radius of the vessel.
iii. Towels or cotton padding and bandaging materials can be wrapped around the patient and then secured with tape.
iv. Approximately 1–2 lbs per square inch of pressure or 25–50 mmHg (3.3–6.7 kPa) pressure should be applied. A blood pressure cuff can be partially inflated and incorporated into the wrap and monitored with the use of a sphygmomanometer. A finger should be easily placed between the wrap and the skin if it is placed appropriately. One pound per square inch is the amount of pressure required to start to see blanching of the tip of your finger.
v. There is a danger of ischemic injury to the structures under the wrap.
vi. The hindlimbs from the toes and the abdomen all the way to the rib cage should be wrapped. Wrapping the hindlimbs prevents pooling of venous blood distal to the wrap and makes sure the bandage is not placed too tightly in the caudal abdomen, possibly occluding the caudal vena cava.
vii. Pain or respiratory distress.
viii. Diaphragmatic movement may have been compromised by placing pressure on the abdomen. By raising blood pressure and increasing venous return to the thorax, intrathoracic wounds are likely to bleed more. If the animal becomes hypertensive, intracranial hemorrhage may worsen.
ix. Diaphragmatic hernia, pneumothorax, hemothorax and severe hemoabdomen causing pressure on the diaphragm.
x. Oxygen supplementation and thoracentesis. Analgesics are required in almost every patient that has counterpressure applied. If this is unsuccessful, the counterpressure can be slowly loosened starting at the cranial aspect of the bandage.
xi. If there is severe chest trauma (pneumothorax, hemothorax, pulmonary contusions), diaphragmatic hernia or intracranial hemorrhage.

124 & 125: Questions

124 A two-year-old, spayed female Cocker Spaniel is presented approximately 1 hour after being hit by a car. Physical examination: temperature – 101.3°F (38.5°C); pulse – 160 bpm; RR – 60 bpm; mucous membranes – gray–pink; CRT – 3 seconds. Blood is noted coming from the right ear canal. Anisocoria with the left pupil larger than the right is seen as well as hyphema in the right eye. The dog is mentally depressed and prefers to lie in lateral recumbency. Comment on the items in the box regarding their therapeutic significance in brain trauma.

Head elevation and position
PCO_2
Hypotension
Hypertension
Jugular vein flow
Hypoxemia
Seizures, hyperthermia
Coughing or gagging
Fluid selection
Osmotic agents
Abdominal counterpressure
Glucocorticoids

125 This 15-week-old, male Rottweiler puppy was presented with a 3-day history of anorexia and vomiting (**125**). He was depressed, febrile (104.1°F, 40.1°C), had increased thick saliva, a prolonged CRT and was tachycardic (180 bpm). He was estimated to be 6–8% dehydrated. There was no localized pain in the abdomen, but he was uncomfortable on palpation. Palpation produced an episode of vomiting. There were no auscultable bowel sounds. Liquid, bloody stool was found on rectal examination. PCV – 38%; TS – 4.9 g/dl; BUN labstick – 30–40 mg/dl; glucose – 120 mg/dl (6.72 mmol/l).

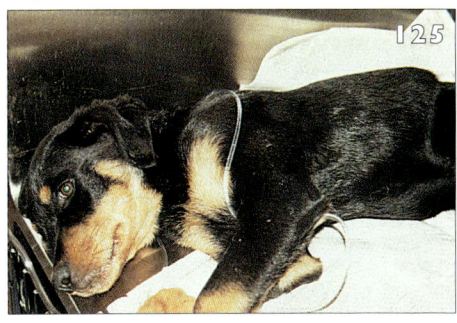

i. Select the best initial fluid plan for this patient:
a. Replace estimated deficit over 4–6 hours with crystalloids, then continue at maintenance plus GI losses.
b. Replace estimated deficit over 4–6 hours with colloids only, then continue with crystalloids at maintenance plus GI losses.
c. Deliver crystalloids at twice maintenance rate to prevent dilution of low serum proteins.
d. Rapid replacement with a combination of crystalloids and colloid until the perfusion parameters normalize.
e. Rapid replacement with hypertonic saline only until perfusion parameters normalize.
ii. Which of the following would not be an indication for systemic antibiotic therapy in this patient:
a. Fever.
b. GI hemorrhage/evidence of loss of mucosal barrier.
c. Marked decrease in auscultable bowel sounds.
d. Suspicion of endotoxemia.
e. Prerenal azotemia on initial data base.
iii. Nutrition is an important part of the treatment plan in any critically ill patient. Is enteral or parenteral feeding preferred in this patient?

124 & 125: Answers

124
- *Head elevation and position.* If the head is below the body, the ICP will increase. If the head is elevated greater than 20° above the body, the MAP can fall, lowering the CPP (CPP = ICP minus MAP). Therefore, the head position for a head trauma patient should be level with the animal or elevated slightly to 20 degrees. In addition to head elevation, the head position should be as normal as possible, allowing free venous flow from the head.
- PCO_2. CO_2 levels that are too high dilate the brain arteries and promote an increase in ICP. If the CO_2 levels are <25 mmHg (<3.3 kPa), the vessels tightly vasoconstrict, and brain flow is impaired. Thus, PCO_2 must be maintained between 30 and 45 mmHg (4.0 and 6.0 kPa).
- *Hypotension.* This can lead to ineffective circulation to the brain and brain tissue hyoxia, worsening secondary brain injury. Hypotension must be aggressively treated and prevented.
- *Hypertension.* This can be as harmful as hypotension. BP that is too high can lead to an increase in ICP. This will then impair cerebral perfusion and lead to cerebral edema. Fluid resuscitation should be done to maintain the systemic MAP between 80 and 100 mmHg (10.6 and 13.3 kPa).
- *Jugular vein flow.* Only three substances live within the bony skull: brain tissue, blood and CSF fluid. When the brain tissue swells, or when there is increased blood flow to the brain, the CSF volume must decrease so that pressure does not increase within the skull. The CSF will empty into the jugular veins, as does some of the blood flow from the head. Obstructing this flow can remove one of the brain's safeguards against increased pressure.
- *Hypoxemia.* Low oxygen tension within the tissues leads to ineffective energy production, consumption of stored energy and inactivation of vital enzyme reactions. The arterial oxygen (PaO_2) must be maintained above 60 mmHg (8.0 kPa) to ensure that there is at least a minimal amount of oxygen available for distribution to the brain tissues.
- *Seizures, hyperthermia.* These complications increase metabolic rate within the brain tissue and contribute to secondary tissue injury.
- *Coughing or gagging.* Both increase ICP, possibly enough in a brain with edema or hemorrhage to cause herniation. Should ventilation be required to maintain the PCO_2 as above, i/v lidocaine is given prior to intubation and extubation to prevent coughing or gagging. In addition, oxygen supplementation by nasal cannula can only be done when the clinician is sure that nasal cannula placement will not cause sneezing.
- *Fluid selection.* Crystalloids are the mainstay of fluid therapy, with normal saline the ideal selection.
- *Osmotic agents.* Agents such as mannitol are used to increase the rheology of the blood. The animal should be maintained iso-osmolar. Furosemide is often administered 30 minutes prior to mannitol to try to offset the increased ICP that can result from mannitol administration.
- *Abdominal counterpressure.* Care must be taken when using this technique for abdominal hemostasis in an animal with head trauma. The increased intra-abdominal pressure can increase ICP by promoting increased venous return from the adbomen and decreasing abdominal and hindlimb blood distribution.
- *Glucocorticoids.* These do not reduce edema in the brain once it has occurred. They have been associated with increased morbidity in humans with brain trauma.

125 i. d.
ii. c, e
iii. Although adequate nutrients can be provided via parenteral nutrition, numerous studies have shown enteral nutrition to be superior to total parenteral feeding. Ideal management would be to provide partial parenteral nutrition and partial enteral nutrition until vomiting is controlled; then maintain on enteral feedings.

126–128: Questions

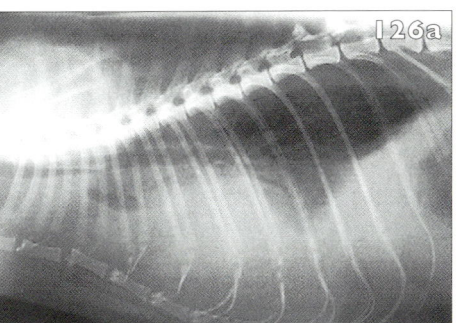
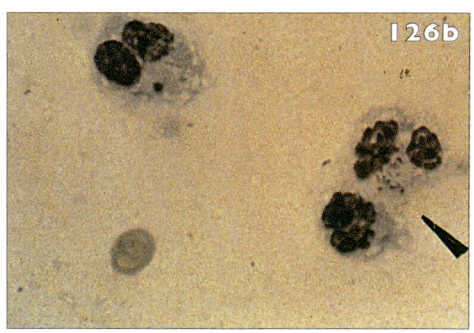

126 A two-year-old, castrated male domestic shorthair cat is presented after 4 days of progressive lethargy, inappetence and increased respiratory effort. Auscultation reveals dull respiratory sounds bilaterally as well as diminished heart sounds. The cat is tachypneic but minimally distressed and stable enough for thoracic radiographs to be taken (**126a**).
i. What is the radiographic diagnosis?
ii. What diagnostic tests would you perform to further characterize the condition?
iii. Describe the findings in this cytology slide (**126b**).
iv. Based on these findings, what type of medical therapy would you initiate, and how would you choose the specific medication?
v. What are your therapeutic options and the advantages of each?

127 An owner presents a cat that has been burned with boiling water within the last half-hour.
i. What are your telephone recommendations to clients with animals that have suffered a thermal burn?
ii. What are the wound closure options for thermal injuries?
iii. What type of dressing would you recommend for thermal injuries?
iv. Discuss fluid therapy for a burn victim.
v. What are some systemic effects of thermal burns?

128 i. What is this instrument (**128**)?
ii. What does it measure and what principle does it use?
iii. Name two uses for this device in the trauma patient with severe degloving injuries to a limb.
iv. Hypotensive resuscitation in the hemorrhaging patient has been said to improve survival if pressures are not normalized until the patient is ready to go to surgery. What is hypotensive resuscitation?

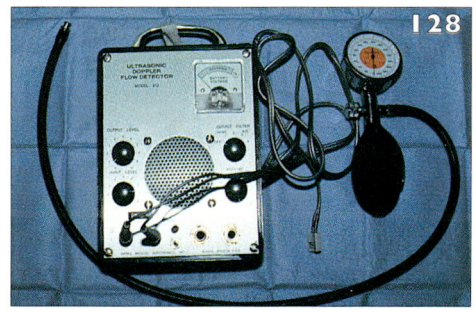

126–128: Answers

126 i. Pleural effusion.
ii. Thoracocentesis and the pleural fluid evaluated for cytologic features, protein concentration and the presence of bacteria.
iii. Degenerate neutrophils predominate (karyorrhectic nuclei, vacuolated cytoplasm) as well as macrophages with intracellular and extracellular bacteria.
iv. Ensure adequate fluid balance and evacuate pleural space. Broad-spectrum, bactericidal i/v antibiotics effective against anaerobes should be started immediately. Fluid should be submitted for aerobic and anaerobic culture and antibiotic sensitivity testing. A Gram stain of the fluid may characterize the bacterial population(s) and guide the choice of an initial antibiotic (consider penicillin G or ampicillin).
v. Tube thoracostomy is more successful at removing thicker exudates and in maintaining a minimal fluid volume in the pleural space. Pleural lavage can be performed to facilitate removal of tenacious debris and dilute bacterial populations; however, this technique has not been proven to improve overall outcome.
 If the history or the cultured bacterial identity is suggestive of a foreign body (e.g. *Nocardia* spp associated with plant awn migration) in the pleural cavity, thoracotomy and open chest pleural lavage is indicated. Pyothorax (empyema) in cats is often caused by penetrating bite or claw wounds.

127 i. The client is told to irrigate the wounded area with cold water for at least 10 minutes. This helps to limit the zone of ischemia. Caution must be employed as systemic hypothermia can occur. Burned animals should be presented to the veterinary hospital immediately.
ii. Complete excision and primary closure; complete excision and autograph, allograph or zenograph; debridement with second intention healing; debridement with delayed grafting.
iii. Dressings, including bandages, biologic dressing and skin grafts, are necessary to prevent desiccation. The primary layer (contact layer) should be adherent, permeable and allow drainage to the secondary absorbent layer. The third layer acts as a protective layer. Non-adherent primary layers are recommended after granulation tissue has formed. Recommended antiseptics are silver nitrate solution or silver sulfadiazine ointment. For a wet to dry bandage, dilute 0.05% chlorhexidine diacetate in water works as an antiseptic.
iv. Isotonic crystalloids (4 ml/kg/%body surface area burned) should be given during the first 24 hours. Half should be given over the first 8 hours, the rest over the following 16 hours. Avoid colloids during the first 8–12 hours (worsens edema formation).
v. Animals with thermal injuries often have a decreased cardiac output, anemia, hypernatremia, hyperkalemia or hypokalemia (later), hypophosphatemia and hypocalcemia. They have an increased risk of acute renal failure, decreased hepatic function and their immune systems are depressed (the primary cause of death in burn patients is infection).

128 i. Doppler blood pressure monitor.
ii. It measures blood flow using the Doppler shift principle. The frequency of waves reflected from moving red cells is shifted slightly relative to the wave that was transmitted from an ultrasonic probe. This is known as the Doppler effect.
iii. Indirect blood pressure monitoring, and assessment of perfusion and the vascular integrity to the distal limb.
iv. The infusion of large amounts of crystalloids to animals with severe uncontrolled hemorrhage has been shown to worsen the outcome in the laboratory animal. In these animals the outcome was improved if fluid resuscitation was provided to maintain a MAP of 60 mmHg (7.8 kPa). In a recent clinical trial, humans with penetrating trauma had improved resuscitation if fluid resuscitation was delayed until the hemorrhage had been surgically controlled.

129–131: Questions

129 This five-year-old female Doberman Pinscher whelped eight puppies 4 weeks ago (**129**). She is febrile (104.9°F, 40.5°C), dehydrated, lethargic and depressed. The left inguinal mammary gland is hard, painful, hot and reddish-purple.

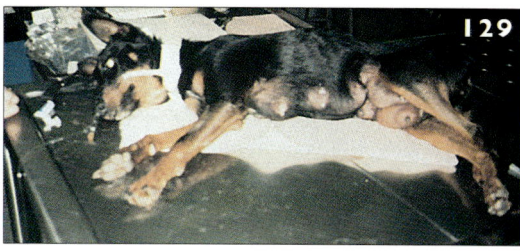

i. What is your tentative diagnosis?
ii. What is your management plan?
iii. What antibiotics have good penetration of the blood–mammary gland barrier and are generally considered safe for nursing offspring?
iv. In cases of mastitis, should the pups always be removed from the dam?

130 This animal was observed being bitten on the head by a rattlesnake (**130**). The owner calls you for advice.
i. What is your recommendation concerning transport?
ii. What are your recommendations concerning first aid?
iii. What do you do to prepare your hospital and staff prior to presentation?

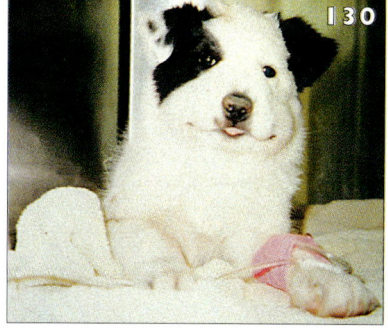

131 A 6-year-old domestic, short-haired cat is presented for labored breathing for 1 day. The lung sounds are louder than normal throughout the thorax. The breathing pattern is smooth, with the chest and abdomen moving in the same direction. There is an intermittent gallop heart sound on auscultation. The lateral thoracic radiograph is shown (**131**). The echo parameters were (normal values in parentheses): left ventricular end-systolic diameter = 4 mm (6–10); left ventricular end-diastolic diameter = 10 mm (11–16);

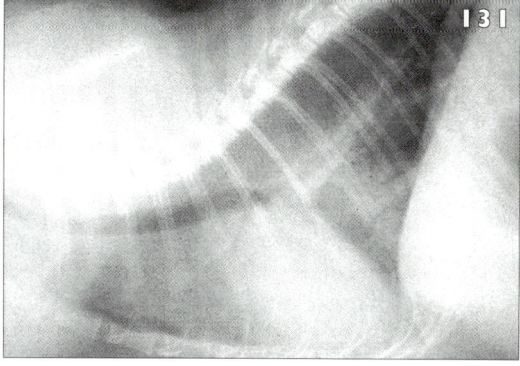

intraventricular septum diastole = 6.2 mm (2.5–5.0); intraventricular septum systole = 11 mm (5–9); left ventricular free wall diastole = 6.8 (2.5–5.00); left ventricular free wall systole = 11 mm (4–9); left atrium systole = 15 mm (8.5–12.5); aortic diastole = 10 mm (6.5–11); Left atrium : Aorta = 1.5 (0.8–1.3); fractional shortening = 60% (29–55%).
i. What is the most likely diagnosis for this cat?
ii. What would you do within the first 30 minutes after presentation?
iii. What long-term medications would you recommend?

129–131: Answers

129 i. Mastitis.
ii. Hospitalize the dam for i/v fluids, bactericidal i/v antibiotics and supportive care. The pups should be removed from the dam and weaned. Warm compresses can be applied to the affected mammary gland to promote drainage. If abscessation, necrosis or gangrene is present, surgical debridement, lancing, flushing and drainage should be performed.
iii. Trimethoprim-sulfa, erythromycin, lincomycin, clindamycin and cephalosporins.
iv. Continued nursing may prevent galactostasis and promote drainage, and is generally safe unless the gland is abscessed or the dam is systemically ill, as in this dog. When pups are allowed to continue nursing, they must be observed for any sign of illness.

130 i. Transport is immediate and respiratory rate and effort monitored.
ii. No first aid other than airway, breathing and hemostasis. Ice therapy, incising over the bite and tourniquets can cause significant tissue damage. Suction 15 minutes after the bite is of no benefit.
iii. Life-threatening problems include airway obstruction, severe shock, hypoxemia, coagulopathy and pyrexia. A tracheostomy set (scalpel blades, small surgical pack, tracheostomy tubes), oxygen and i/v fluids should be prepared.

131 i. Hypertrophic cardiomyopathy.
ii. Oxygen; i/v furosemide at 2–7 mg/kg; sedative if necessary; 0.25inch nitroglycerine paste rubbed into the skin on a clipped area; minimize stress.
iii. Compliance of the ventricles can be improved with either beta-blockers such as atenolol or calcium channel blockers such as diltiazem. These drugs can decrease the heart rate as well. Angiotensin-converting enzyme inhibitors (enalapril, benazepril or captopril) are used for afterload reduction.

132–134: Questions

132 A nine-year-old Miniature Schnauzer presents with a 3-day history of vomiting. The dog is febrile and shows signs of shock (weak, hyperemic mucous membranes, rapid RR, tachycardia and weak pulses). Based on history, physical examination and laboratory findings, a presumptive diagnosis of pancreatitis is made.

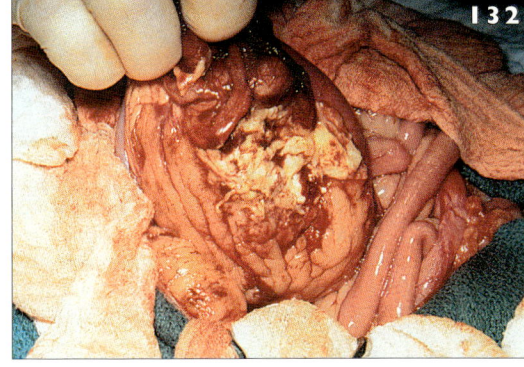

i. What are the general indications for surgical exploration in pancreatitis?
ii. The pancreas is shown (**132**). What is the most likely pathology of this gland? How can this be treated surgically? Describe the procedure.
iii. What criteria are used to determine if the abdomen should be left open? How should a pancreas be drained postoperatively?
iv. What options are available for postoperative feeding? What are the pros and cons of enteral versus parenteral feeding? Should a specific type of diet be chosen and, if yes, what type?

133 This five-year-old, female Cocker Spaniel presented for evaluation of decreased appetite (**133**). PCV – 38%; TS – 6.8 gm/dl; ACT – 90 seconds; platelet count – 65,000/µl.
i. What abnormality is seen here?
ii. Abnormalitites of which part of the coagulation system will result in these clinical signs?
iii. Is the platelet count low enough to result in clinical signs of spontaneous hemorrhage?
iv. Name four categories for the etiology of the coagulation abnormality. List one example for each cause.

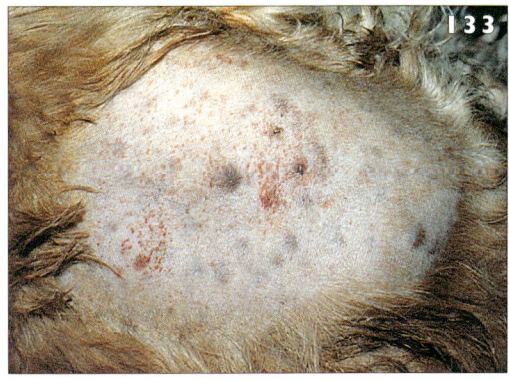

134 A three-year-old dog was witnessed ingesting a package of material 2 days earlier. Now the dog presents with a history of vomiting, depression, anorexia, polydipsia, polyuria and diarrhea. Serum chemistry reveals a very high total calcium (18 mg/dl [4.5 mmol/l]) (normal 8–10 mg/dl [2–2.5 mmol/l]).
i. What toxin is likely to have been ingested by this dog?
ii. What are the major organ systems affected by the hypercalcemia?
iii. What are the specific treatments for this toxin?

132–134: Answers

132 i. Trauma, peritonitis, pancreatic mass (abscess/phlegmon, tumour), patient that is not responding to medical therapy.
ii. The pancreas appears to be suppurative with abscessed necrotic tissue present. This will require surgical debridement. All powder should be removed from gloves because it is extremely irritating to the pancreas. The viability of the pancreas is assessed by noting the color of the organ as well as evidence of a patent vascular supply. Adhesions should be gently broken down. The pancreas is lavaged and white areas or necrotic avascular areas should be debrided. If in doubt, the pancreas is lavaged again. The capsule of the pancreas is incised with a #15 blade and hemostats are used to dissect between lobules. The affected area is cross-clamped and ligated with 4-0 monofilament suture (ideally polypropylene or polybutester). Bipolar electrosurgery can also be used to debride. The pancreatic ducts are ligated. The capsule is closed as required with a simple continuous pattern using the same suture material. If the bile duct is obstructed, a cholecystoduodenostomy may be required. If pyloric or duodenal obstructions are present due to non-resectable fibrous tissue, diversion procedures such as gastroduodenostomy or gastrojejunostomy may be required. The abdomen is extensively lavaged with warm saline. If the abdomen is going to be left open, the falciform fat and most of the omentum will need to be removed.
iii. If a suppurative peritonitis was found, the abdomen should be left open. Suction or sump drains should be placed adjacent to the pancreas and the abdomen closed or left open as required. The drains may need to be tacked to the serosa with a small suture. When the drain is removed, gentle traction is applied which will cause the tacking suture to pull out from the serosa.
iv. Enteral nutrition with a monomeric diet can be fed if a jejunostomy tube is placed. Enteral feeding into the stomach and duodenum should be avoided until signs of pancreatitis have resolved. Parenteral nutrition can be used, although lipid should probably be avoided until signs of pancreatitis resolve.

133 i. Evidence of petechiae.
ii. The presence of petechiae suggests the presence of either a vascular or platelet abnormality (vasculitis, thrombocytopenia, thrombocytopathia).
iii. No. If the platelet count is less than $40,000/\mu l$, the animal may have a bleeding tendency. Spontaneous hemorrhage, however, does not usually occur until the platelet count is less than $20,000/\mu l$.
iv. Causes of thrombocytopenia are decreased platelet production (myeloproliferative disease), consumption (DIC), sequestration (liver/spleen disease) or destruction (immune-mediated disease)

134 i. A cholecalciferol containing rodenticide.
ii. The central nervous, cardiovascular, GI and renal systems.
iii. 0.9% saline i/v to induce diuresis; furosemide (2–5 mg/kg every 8–12 hours); oral prednisolone (2 mg/kg every 12 hours); salmon calcitonin (4–6 IU/kg every 2–3 hours); peritoneal dialysis.

135–137: Questions

135 On the morning of a beautiful summer day, a five-year-old, male German Pointer played unattended in the backyard garden. During the following 24 hours the right side of the dog's face became swollen (135). The dog developed urticaria and became lethargic, unable to walk and vomited several times.
i. What is your presumptive diagnosis?
ii. What pathologic mechanism(s) is involved?
iii. What is the treatment protocol?
iv. Which clinical signs would you expect if it were a cat?

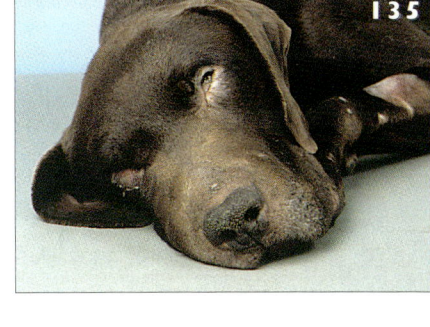

136 As you finally find time to cook your supper and sit down to eat, your triage nurse alerts you that a poorly perfused intact female dog, which is leaking a malodorous seropurulent discharge from her vulva, has arrived at the hospital (136a). A decision is made to reperfuse the patient over a short time period and surgically remove an infected uterus. During surgical exploration an inflamed peritonitis with seropurulent peritoneal fluid leaking from the fallopian tubes is discovered along with an inflamed and pus-filled uterus (136b).
i. What is the best surgical treatment for a septic peritonitis?
ii. What is the plan for managing this treatment option?
iii. When and how do you decide to complete this treatment?

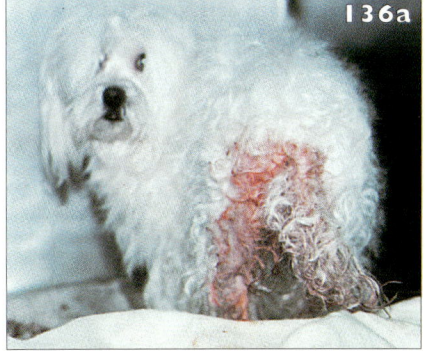

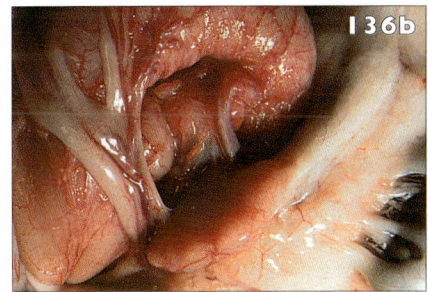

137 An adult dog with a gastric dilatation/volvulus is presented for emergency surgery. Following i/v fluids, oxygen supplementation, glucocorticoid administration and ECG assessment, a percutaneous puncture of the distended stomach was done to relieve the gastric tympani.
i. What concerns do you have regarding selection of anesthetic agents for this dog?
ii. What anesthetic agents would you use?

135–137: Answers

135 i. Angioedema or anaphylaxis, probably caused by an insect sting. Anaphylaxis can be 'localized anaphylaxis' (urticaria and angioedema) or 'systemic anaphylaxis' (generalized signs). In the above case the generalized signs should indicate that the disease is systemic.
ii. Immediate type I hypersensitivity reaction.
iii. The offending agent is removed if possible and supportive care given with antihistamines, corticosteroids and epinephrine as indicated. The patient is best hospitalized for 12–24 hours for observation for further delayed or protracted reactions.
iv. Early signs in cats are different from those in dogs. Extreme pruritus of the head and respiratory distress due to upper airway obstruction by laryngeal edema, bronchoconstriction and increased mucus production are common.

136 i. Providing an open drainage of the infected peritoneal cavity is the best treatment of a septic peritonitis. The infected source and devitalized tissue need to be removed and a culture and sensitivity of the tissue performed. Removal of the falciform fat and either removal or tacking of the omentum is required to prevent them from obstructing the opening. Copious warm saline lavage and suction is required, followed by placement of a loose zipper closure in the external fascia of the rectus abdominus involving the area from the xiphoid to mid-way between the umbilicus and pubis. If not infected, the tissues of the remaining incision can be closed primarily. Multiple layers of sterile laparotomy pads or towels are used to cover the closure, followed by a drape and bandage.
ii. Collection of the drainage fluid with sterile laparotomy pads or towels and replacement of the towels as they become soaked with peritoneal drainage, or at least every 24 hours. The patient will also require appropriate medical therapy including fluid support, oncotic support, antibiotics, analgesics and nutrition.
iii. At least 72 hours of open drainage is usually required. After this point, as the drainage decreases, an assessment is made regarding appropriate closure. When closure is performed, the middle of the zipper is cut and the two ends tightened and tied, closing the body wall. The deep subcutaneous tissues (which have started to develop a granulation bed) and skin can be closed in a single layer of mattress sutures.

137 i. Refrain from using cardiovascular depressant anesthetic drugs (i.e. do not use or limit use of vasodilators such as acepromazine, thiobarbiturates, halothane, etc). Do not use nitrous oxide. Isoflurane is vasodilatory, requiring low flow anesthesia, adequate volume resuscitation and careful BP monitoring.
ii. Preferably use potent opiates such as fentanyl combined with sedatives like droperidol or diazepam with mandatory artificial ventilation. Intermittent bolus anesthesia with these agents can be successful in the very cardiovascularly compromised patient. If the cardiovascular system is stable, induction with these agents and careful maintenance on isoflurane is acceptable. Ketamine/diazepam combination would be another acceptable inducing plan. There must be ECG monitoring for cardiac arrhythmias.

138–140: Questions

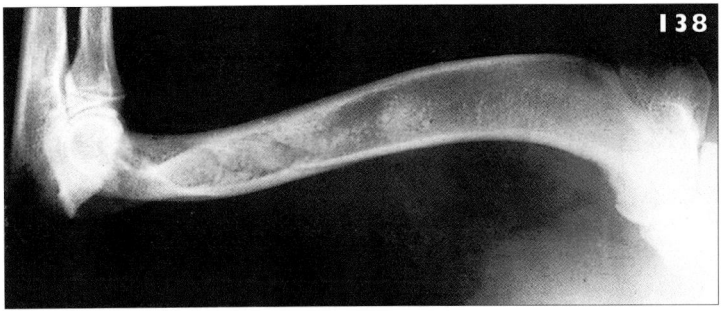

138 This seven-month-old, male German Shepherd Dog started to become acutely lame on its right forelimb 5 days ago (**138**). The dog was presented as an emergency because of acute exacerbation in this limb. On physical examination the dog had a rectal temperature of 103.6°F (39.8°C); he was reluctant to stand and was only toe touching with his right forelimb once he did stand; no obvious external trauma could be seen. Orthopedic examination revealed no obvious skeletal fractures. Deep palpation of the left proximal ulna and the shaft of the right humerus was painful. Radiographs of the right humerus were taken.
i. What is your radiographic interpretation, and what are your differentials at this time?
ii. What is the treatment of this problem?
iii. What is the prognosis ?

139 i. Major blood vessels, such as both external jugular veins, may need to be ligated to control hemorrhage. Name eight other major vessels that can be ligated without causing permanent vascular compromise to the patient (assuming no damage to collateral circulatory pathways).
ii. The caudal abdominal aorta can be ligated caudal to what organ without causing permanent vascular compromise to the patient (assuming no damage to collateral circulatory pathways)?
iii. The caudal abdominal vena cava can be ligated caudal to what organ without causing permanent vascular compromise to the patient (assuming no damage to collateral circulatory pathways)?

140 A cat presented with a sudden onset of labored breathing. A diaphragmatic hernia was confirmed on radiographs and there was a partially filled stomach in the thoracic cavity. You decided to perform a surgical repair of the hernia after initial stabilization of the cat. What were the principal complicating factors concerning the anesthesia of this cat?

138–140: Answers

138 i. Increased focal intramedullary densities that are very suspicious of panosteitis; this should be your working diagnosis. Differentials also include osteomyelitis and hypertrophic osteodystrophy.
ii. Rest and pain control with NSAIDs. Recommendations include buffered aspirin (10–20 mg/kg p/o tid). Side-effects of prolonged aspirin use include GI ulceration with vomiting and diarrhea, and altered platelet function. If NSAIDs are given over a prolonged period of time, misoprostol, a synthetic prostaglandin E_1 analog, should be added (2–5g/kg p/o tid) for the same period of time. Other choices of NSAIDs include phenylbutazolidine, ibuprofen and flunixin meglumine products. Similar, sometimes stronger side-effects are observed with these drugs. Steroids are not recommended.
iii. Excellent. It is important to educate the owner about the progression of this disease. Clinical signs can be present until the age of 20 months, usually more than one limb is affected and the lameness shifts from one limb to the other. Pain relief should only be considered during the periods of lameness to diminish possible side-effects.

139 i. Both common carotid arteries; both brachiocephalic veins; both subclavian veins; both brachial arteries; both brachial veins; both cephalic veins; both femoral arteries; both external iliac arteries; both common iliac veins; and both femoral veins.
ii. The kidney.
iii. The liver.

140 Increased risk of developing an aspiration pneumonia; limited expansion of the lungs (low tidal volume) making artificial ventilation with 100% oxygen mandatory; high inspiratory pressures which will limit venous return and decrease cardiac output; possible trauma-induced contusion of lung and/or heart leading to an increased risk of pulmonary edema and cardiac arrhythmias.

141 & 142: Questions

141 This dog presented for a dog bite wound on his dorsal thorax which required sutures (**141**).
i. What are the indications for drain placement?
ii. What are some likely pathogens of a dog bite wound?
iii. What criteria should be used to determine whether a wound should be closed primarily or left open to heal?
iv. How might this wound progress to sepsis or septic shock?
v. What should be done after a Penrose drain has been placed surgically?
vi. Discuss the proper removal of a Penrose drain.

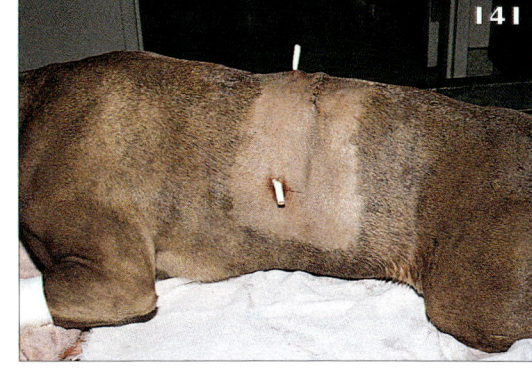

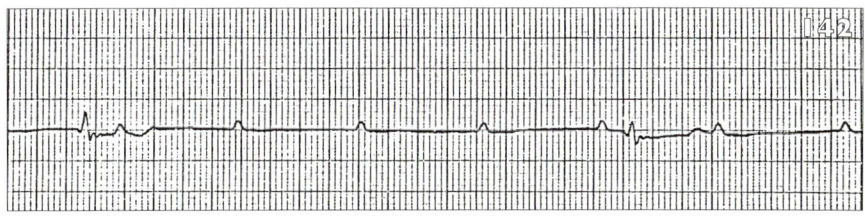

142 A 12-year-old, castrated male Dachshund presents after a 'seizure-like' episode. He is nervous but ambulatory on presentation. He is bradycardic and a grade II/VI systolic murmur is auscultated over the left apex.
i. What is the ECG diagnosis (**142**)?
ii. What are possible causes of the abnormality?
iii. What treatment options do you offer the owner?

141 & 142: Answers

141 i. Obliteration of dead space, elimination of fluid accumulation and prophylactic prevention of fluid or air accumulation.
ii. *Streptococcus* spp, *Staphylococcus* spp, *Pasteurella* spp, *E. coli*, *Pseudomonas* spp and *Proteus* spp. Hospital acquired bacteria are typically *Pseudomonas* spp, *Klebsiella* spp and *Proteus* spp. Anaerobes involved are *Bacteroides* spp and *Clostridium perfringens*.
iii. Primary closure is appropriate if the wound can be converted to a clean wound with debridement and lavage; when there is no significant tension on the wound when the skin is closed; if the wound is not associated with a crush injury; if it is not infected ($<10^5$ bacteria/gram of tissue on quantitative count; if it does not contain beta hemolytic streptococci, hemolytic *E. coli*, *Pseudomonas* spp, *Staphylococcus* spp or an anaerobe; if is not a puncture wound (non-dissecting puncture wounds should be opened by inserting a hemostat and opening the blades rather than closing the wound).
iv. There is a risk of spread of infection through the fascial planes if there is not adequate debridement, lavage and drainage. Sepsis occurs when bacteria get into the blood stream.
v. An absorbent bandage should be applied over both ends of the drain. It should be applied with light compression to minimize dead space.
vi. The skin surrounding the ends of the drain should be cleansed thoroughly and rinsed well. Retention sutures are removed and traction is applied to both ends of the drain. The drain is stretched until a portion that was previously covered is exposed. The drain is severed through this exposed area and the two portions are removed so that none of the previously exposed drain enters the wound tract.

142 i. Third degree atrioventricular (AV) block. Ventricular rate 40 bpm.
ii. Idiopathic, myocarditis, fibrosis, Lyme disease.
iii. Medical therapy may be attempted. Propantheline bromide, an anticholinergic, has been used in incomplete AV block, though is not likely to be effective if an i/v dose of atropine proves to be ineffective. Bronchodilators, e.g. aminophylline or terbutaline, are sympathomimetic and may increase HR. Both of these drugs must be used with extreme caution in patients with congestive heart failure or cardiomyopathy. Ultimately, pacemaker implantation is advised.

143–145: Questions

143 A newly acquired four-month-old Miniature Poodle presented with sudden onset pain of some 20 hours' duration. There was blepharospasm and excessive lacrimation, and the puppy had been constantly rubbing the eye (143). These features had been noticed after the household cat and the puppy had exchanged social niceties!
i. Describe the pathology seen in the eye.
ii. What is your diagnosis?
iii. What treatment would you prescribe?
iv. Given the likely etiology, what complications must be ruled out?

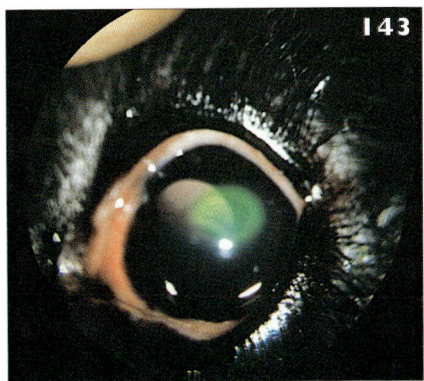

144 The following questions are directed toward the acute management of an animal that has experienced a severe traumatic injury.
i. Define primary survey. What is assessed during this?
ii. Define secondary survey. What is assessed during this?
iii. List at least eight catastrophic complications of trauma that could cause an injured animal to be 'dying before your eyes'.
iv. What should be done as an immediate life-saving procedure for a traumatized animal that is barrel chested; has rapid, choppy breathing with little chest wall movement; has no lung sounds auscultated bilaterally; is cyanotic; and is in severe decompensatory shock?
v. In general, when a traumatized animal has difficulty breathing or some signs of shock, what is the first intervention that should be done?
vi. The animal has been given what would appear to the normal clinician to be an adequate volume of fluids. However, the signs of shock persist. List at least ten reasons for shock to be unresponsive to initial fluid infusion.
vii. How can the adequacy of volume replacement be assessed?
viii. It is recommended that patients that have experienced trauma be hospitalized for a minimum of 12–24 hours to observe for complications that may not be apparent on presentation. Name some of the complications that have a delayed onset of clinical signs.

145 A 12-year-old Irish Setter is presented as an emergency for inspiratory stridor. A presumptive diagnosis of laryngeal paralysis is made; the patient needs to be anesthetized for tracheal cannulation.
i. Which complicating factors need to be considered?
ii. What would be your anesthetic approach?

143–145: Answers

143 i. The use of fluorescein is routine in the differential diagnosis of anterior segment pain; in this instance a central area of epithelial loss was demonstrated.
ii. Corneal ulceration of probable traumatic origin (cat scratch).
iii. Routine therapy should include the use of a topical antibiotic and an Elizabethan collar. Atropine might be indicated if ciliary and iris spasm are suspected, and collagenase inhibitors could be used if the ulcer rapidly gains depth over the next 12 hours.
iv. In the absence of infection this type of ulcer should repair rapidly, but cat scratches always involve the potential complication of corneal penetration. A careful examination is required to rule out this possibility.

144 i. Primary survey is the immediate and rapid evaluation of a patient for life-threatening problems. Airway, breathing, bleeding, circulation, consciousness and neurologic deficits are assessed.
ii. Secondary survey is the more thorough and timely assessment of the patient for complications and injuries. This would include abdominal palpation, evaluation of the skin and musculoskeletal systems, eyes, ears, throat and other physical parameters.
iii. Airway obstruction or injury; cardiopulmonary arrest; internal hemorrhage; external hemorrhage; cardiac tamponade; tension pneumothorax; open pneumothorax; malignant arrhythmias; brain stem injury; financial constraints of the owner.
iv. The physical signs described are most compatible with a tension pneumothorax. An incision should be made rapidly into the chest wall to allow the accumulated free air in the pleural space that is under tension to escape.
v. Oxygen.
vi. The volume of fluids infused were insufficient to provide adequate intravascular filling; fluids infused were adequate but there is an ongoing loss through hemorrhage, vomiting, diarrhea, third body fluid spacing; severe pain; bradyarrhythmia; tachyarrhythmia; hypoglycemia; severe electrolyte disorders such as hypomagnesemia, hypokalemia, hyperkalemia, hypophosphatemia; severe acid–base disturbances; excessive vasodilation; excessive vasoconstriction; inadequate cardiac function; organ ischemia; brain dysfunction; tension pneumothorax; pericardial tamponade; impaired venous return.
vii. In the ideal situation a pulmonary artery catheter would be placed and the pulmonary capillary wedge pressure and cardiac output would be determined. However, in the more typical private practice setting, CVP will suffice, monitoring the trend of change during and after fluid infusion. The goal is to bring the CVP up to 6–8 cmH_2O (3.8–5.1 kPa).
viii. Ongoing blood loss; pneumothorax; brain concussion; hairline fractures; muscle and tendon injuries; ruptured urinary bladder; ruptured biliary tract; avulsed mesenteric vessel; cardiac arrhythmias; pericardial tamponade; lung contusions.

145 i. Hyperthermia, hypovolemia, hypoxemia, airway edema and secretions, and secondary pulmonary edema.
ii. An anesthetic approach should include: establishing i/v line for fluid replacement therapy; administration of supplemental oxygen; swift induction of anesthesia (choices include propofol, methohexital or ketamine/diazepam) followed by endotracheal intubation and 100% oxygen; normalize body temperature.

146–148: Questions

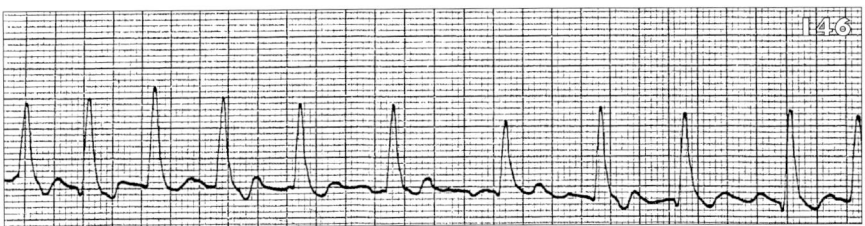

146 This ECG (146) was recorded from a ten-year-old, castrated male Golden Retriever presented with a 1-week history of anorexia and productive cough. On physical examination he was dyspneic with crackles over all lung fields and he had moderate abdominal distension
i. What is the arrhythmia present?
ii. With what conditions is this rhythm commonly associated?
iii. What is the next essential diagnostic test you would perform?
iv. What should your initial treatment of this patient include?

147 i. What is your radiographic diagnosis (147)?
ii. What blood gas abnormality would you expect in this patient?
iii. What would be the fluid of choice for initial fluid resuscitation?
iv. What drug would be contraindicated to control vomiting in this patient?
v. Given the diagnosis of gastric outflow obstruction, how would you expect the owner to describe the vomitus in terms of appearance, effort and timing in relation to eating?

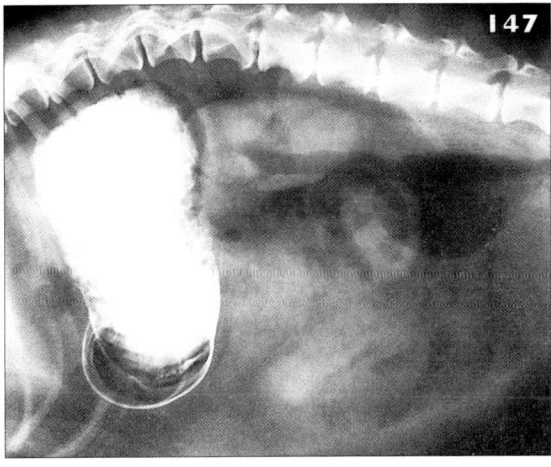

148 A 4.5 kg Poodle has eaten a lot of baker's chocolate.
i. What signs will the dog exhibit if it has ingested a toxic dose?
ii. What is the mechanism of action of chocolate?
iii. What are the major organ systems affected by the methylxanthines?
iv. What are the specific treatments for chocolate intoxication?

146–148: Answers

146 i. Atrial fibrillation with a ventricular rate of 200–220 bpm.
ii. Dilated cardiomyopathy is most likely present. Other conditions commonly associated with atrial fibrillation are chronic atrioventricular valvular disease (particularly advanced mitral regurgitation) and occasionally in dogs lacking other evidence of cardiac disease, cardiac trauma, gastric dilatation or electrolyte abnormalities.
iii. Chest radiographs and an echocardiogram can be performed once the heart failure treatment has been initiated and the patient is more stable.
iv. The cardiac failure state requires the use of furosemide and vasodilators (enalapril – 0.5 mg/kg sid or 0.25 mg/kg bid) to improve cardiac output. It is not necessary to convert atrial fibrillation to a normal sinus rhythm, but the goal is to reduce the ventricular response with digoxin by slowing conduction through the atrioventricular node. A beta-blocker or calcium channel blocker may be added at a later date to further decrease the ventricular rate. Contractility can be improved rapidly by administration of dobutamine (5–10 µg/kg/minute) by CRI.

147 i. Gastric outflow obstruction.
ii. Hypochloremic, metabolic alkalosis.
iii. 0.9% NaCl. If chloride is provided by the i/v administration of saline, excess bicarbonate is eliminated in the urine to correct the metabolic alkalosis
iv. Metoclopramide is contraindicated in gastric outflow obstruction.
v. A white mucoid fluid, or containing undigested food if occurring soon after eating. The vomiting would be quite forceful and possibly described as projectile.

148 i. Vomiting, polydipsia, polyuria, restlessness, hyperactivity, tachycardia, tachypnea, ataxia, muscle tremors, seizures, cardiac arrhythmias and even death.
ii. Chocolate contains methylxanthines which inhibit phosphodiesterase, cause release of catecholamines, competitively inhibit adenosine receptors and increase myocyte intracellular calcium.
iii. The neuromuscular, cardiovascular and central nervous systems are the major sites of action of the methylxanthines and chocolate toxicity.
iv. Activated charcoal (0.5 g/kg every 3 hours for 72 hours). Diazepam or barbiturate to control seizures. Control arrhythmias with lidocaine (ventricular) or beta-blockers. Place a urinary catheter or keep the urinary bladder drained to prevent reabsorption of the toxin.

149 & 150 Questions

149 A four-year-old, castrated male mixed-breed dog (35 kg) was presented after being hit by a car (149). Physical and neurologic examination found the following problems: middle stage of shock; labored, choppy breathing with no lungs auscultable on the left side; gray gum color; significant distress and anxiety; posterior paresis with deep pain and voluntary motor activity present on neurologic examination. The dog has received flow-by oxygen

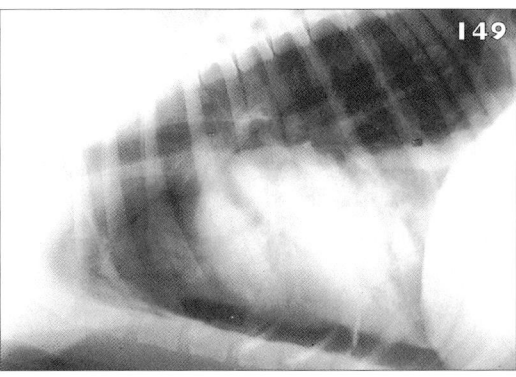

and has a peripheral catheter and rapid infusion of crystalloids. A thoracocentesis of the left side finds no negative pressure. A chest tube is placed on the left side and continuous suction employed. However, the dog still shows labored breathing and has poor gum color. He has been given hetastarch, glucocorticoids and a first generation cephalosporin i/v. His arterial blood gases are as follows: FiO_2 – 40%; PaO_2 – 54 mmHg (7.2 kPa); $PaCO_2$ – 56 mmHg (7.5 kPa); pH – 7.35; HCO_3 – 28 mEq/l.
i. What is your blood gas diagnosis?
ii. What is your therapeutic option at this time?
iii. What are the initial ventilator settings for the following parameters:
a. FiO_2 (fraction of inspired oxygen).
b. Respiratory rate.
c. Tidal volume.
d. End-expiratory pressure.
e. Inspiratory:expiratory ratio.
f. Inspiratory pressure.
g. Mode of ventilation (assisted versus controlled).
   After ventilation was initated, the chest was auscultated and there was no air movement on the right side. In addition, the end-tidal CO_2 monitor showed a $PaCO_2$ of 68 mmHg (9.0 kPa).
iv. What should be done now?
   The dog has now been on the ventilator for 6 hours. A repeat arterial blood gas showed: PaO_2 – 150 mmHg (20 kPa); $PaCO_2$ – 70 mmHg (9.3 kPa); pH – 7.25; HCO_3 – 30 mEq/l.
v. What should be assessed and adjusted to try to alleviate the acute respiratory acidosis in this dog?
   The carbon dioxide level has now been lowered, but the PaO_2 is still inadequate on 100% oxygen. The PaO_2 is 150 mmHg (20 kPa) and the shunt fraction is 150 (<200 is suggestive of intrapulmonary shunting).
vi. What can be done to try to improve this oxygenation problem?

150 A dog has been receiving aspirin daily for arthritic hips during the last several months. Two days ago he received an injection of corticosteroids for a flea allergic dermatitis. He started vomiting blood and his stool became tarry black.
i. What is the most likely cause of this dog's problem given the above history?
ii. What are the major organs affected by these drugs during intoxication?
iii. What is the mechanism of action of these drugs?
iv. What are the specific treatments for this intoxication?

149 & 150 Answers

149 i. Partially compensated respiratory acidosis and hypoxemia (low shunt fraction).
ii. Ventilator therapy with 100% oxygen.
iii. a – 1.0 (100%); b – 10–12 bpm; c – 7–10 ml/kg = 7×35 = 245–350 ml as measured at the endotracheal tube of the dog; d – 2–5 cm H_2O (1.3–3.2 kPa); e – 1:2; f – 25–30 cm H_2O (15.8–19.0 kPa); g – controlled (mandatory).
iv. A chest tube should be place in the right hemithorax and the tube maintained with continuous suction.
v. Increase the ventilatory rate; increase tidal volume; check the endotracheal tube for kinking or obstruction with secretions; decrease the dead space in the ventilator and in the patient; treat any fever or seizure or other metabolic disturbance that might increase CO_2 production; make sure the exhalation valve is working and that the dog is not rebreathing his CO_2; minimize dead space.
vi. Increase the positive end-expiratory pressure to between 5 and 10 cm H_2O (3.2 and 6.3 kPa) as directed by the blood gases.

150 i. The most likely cause of this dog's clinical signs is gastric ulceration secondary to administration of an NSAID as well as a corticosteroid. Each drug alone has the potential to cause gastric ulceration. When combined, these drugs are even more potent in causing gastric ulceration.
ii. The renal and GI systems.
iii. Corticosteroids have a variety of effects, but specifically in this case they maintain cellular membranes and prevent the liberation of arachidonic acid from the cell membranes. This is a key step in the production of prostaglandins. The NSAID inhibits cyclooxygenase which is another enzyme involved in the production of prostaglandins. Prostaglandins in the stomach help protect the gastric mucosa against ulceration while vasodilatory prostaglandins help maintain renal vasodilation, particularly during hypotensive states. Diminished production of these prostaglandins may result in gastric ulceration and renal ischemia.
iv. Histamine receptor H_2 antagonists, sucralfate, misoprostol (a prostaglandin analog), ± whole blood transfusion, ± antiemetics, i/v fluids, ± dopamine and diuretics.

151 & 152: Questions

151 A female ferret of unknown age is presented for acute onset of severe lethargy (151). The owners obtained the pet 2 weeks ago from an elementary school class which had owned the ferret for 6 years. It is not known if the animal has been spayed. Physical examination reveals a mentally depressed thin ferret. HR – 200 bpm; mucous membranes – pale pink; CRT – 1 second; spleen is enlarged but no masses are palpated. Blood glucose registers 'Lo' on the glucometer.
i. What is the presumptive diagnosis?
ii. Which one of the following is NOT a mechanism by which glucocorticoids increase serum blood glucose?
a. Increasing hepatic glycogen.
b. Decreasing the uptake and use of glucose by peripheral tissues.
c. Permissive effect on glucagon and catecholamines.
d. Decreasing receptor sensitivity to insulin.
iii. Diazoxide acts by:
a. Increasing glycogenolysis and gluconeogenesis.
b. Promoting glucagon and growth hormone release.
c. Inhibiting insulin release.
d. a and c.
e. b and c.

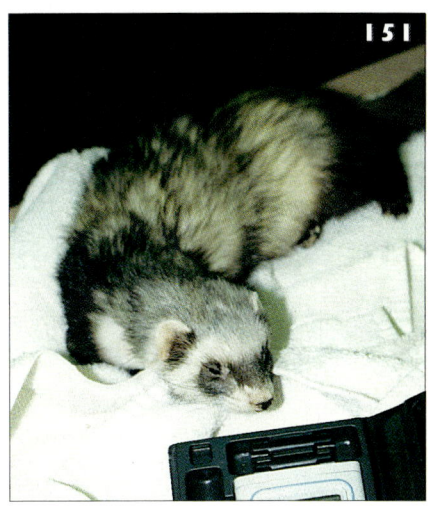

iv. A definitive diagnosis of an insulinoma can be obtained by:
a. Repeatable fasting hypoglycemia.
b. Elevated absolute insulin levels.
c. Exploratory surgery and histopathology.
d. b and c.
e. All of the above.

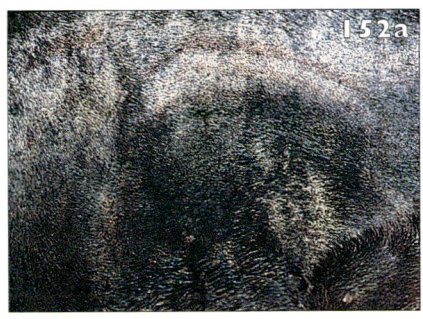
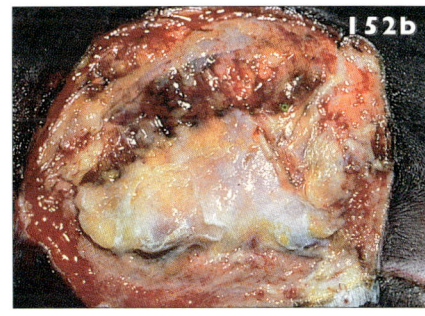

152 The left thoracic wall of a two-year-old Miniature Pinscher that was trapped behind a refrigerator and was burned by the cooling element is shown (152a). Several days later dead skin was removed surgically (152b).
i. What first aid could be given by the owner?
ii. How are burns generally classified in veterinary medicine?
iii. Why are burn victims susceptible to infections, sepsis and septic shock?
iv. What bacteria are found in burn victims, and what is their origin?

151 & 152: Answers

151 i. Insulinoma.
ii. d.
iii. d.
iv. d

152 i. Separate the patient from the burning agent. Flush and cool affected areas with copious amounts of cool water for 10–15 minutes. Support breathing if necessary by mouth-to-nose resuscitation. Dry patient and wounds carefully with a clean (preferably sterile) towel to prevent the development of hypothermia. Wrap the patient in a clean sheet and use an additional blanket to avoid chilling. Transport the pateint as quickly as possible to the veterinary critical care facility.
ii. The severity of a burn injury is determined based on three characteristics:
The degree of depth. Superficial burns have only part of the epidermis involved and are very painful, thickened, erythematous and desquamated. Superficial partial burns involve part of the epidermis and the mid-dermis and they are characterized by less pain, erythema and subcutaneous edema. Deep partial burns involve the entire epidermis and part of the dermis and are almost painless, dry and do not blanche. Full thickness burns involve the entire thickness of the skin and are characterized by the absence of pain, severe subcutaneous edema and blanched or charred and leather-like skin.
The extent of the injury. This is expressed as a percentage of the total body surface area (TBSA). A rapid method of estimating the extent of a burn is the 'rule of nine': each forelimb 9%, each hindlimb 18%, head and neck 9%, dorsal and ventral thorax/abdomen each 18%.
The location of the injury. Burns including parts of the extremities and head are considered more severe.
iii. Suppression of humoral and cell-mediated immunity occurs in major burn patients, beginning when 20% or more of the TBSA is burned. Furthermore, burn wounds offer optimal conditions for bacterial colonization. Apart from impaired defensive mechanisms because of insufficient local circulation, they offer microorganisms an ideal moist and protien-rich environment.
iv. *Staphylococcus intermedius* and *Streptococcus* spp are the first to colonize the wound. They originate from the normal flora of the skin, respiratory tract and GI tract. Endogenous and exogenous coliforms and *Pseudomonas* spp follow in several days. Nosocomial infections with resistant organisms are a potential hazard, making aseptic procedures mandatory.

153–155: Questions

153 An eight-year-old, 18.5 kg, castrated male Boxer presented with acute onset shaking, abdominal splinting and hematemesis (**153**). PCV – 46%; TS – 6.9 g/l; platelet count – 3×10^9/l; sodium – 169 mEq/l; potassium – 4.1 mEq/l; chloride – 121 mEq/l. Urea and creatinine were normal. During the first 6 hours of hospitalization the dog was noted to be polyuric and mildly hematuric. Urine SG was 1.008, with an associated 1.0 kg weight loss, and sodium was 190 mmol/l. The dog was considered to be 8% dehydrated at presentation.

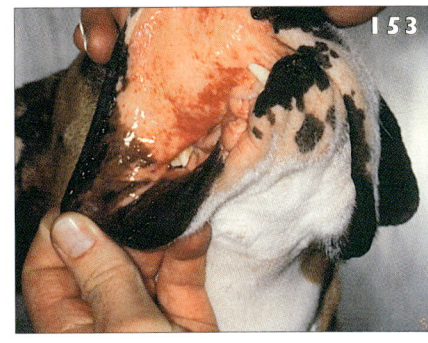

i. Calculate the fluid deficit and select a replacement solution.
ii. List causes of hypernatremia.
iii. Six hours after admission, calculate the amount of water to be administered (lost). What solution would be appropriate at this time?

154 A ten-year-old, castrated male Beagle presents with an acute onset of respiratory distress and collapse. On presentation he is severely dyspneic, mucous membranes are cyanotic and crackles are auscultated diffusely over the left and right lung fields. A high-pitched grade IV/VI holosystolic murmur is present over the left apex, HR is 124 bpm and femoral pulses are weak.
i. What are your differential diagnoses?
ii. What do your immediate interventions include for this patient?
iii. Two hours later, the dog appears more

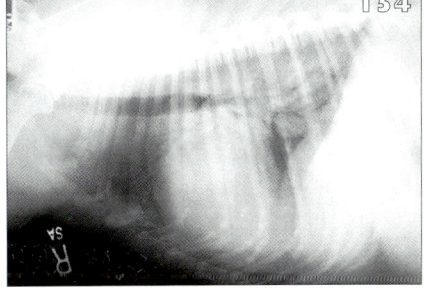

stable and you obtain thoracic radiographs. What are your differential considerations now?
iv. How do the physical examination and radiographic findings (**153**) support your tentative diagnosis?

155 This one-year-old cat had three healthy kittens (**155**). Following parturition, the owners noticed a large red mass protruding from the vagina.
i. What is your diagnosis?
ii. What is your management plan?
iii. What serious, life-threatening complication may result from this problem, and how can it be managed?

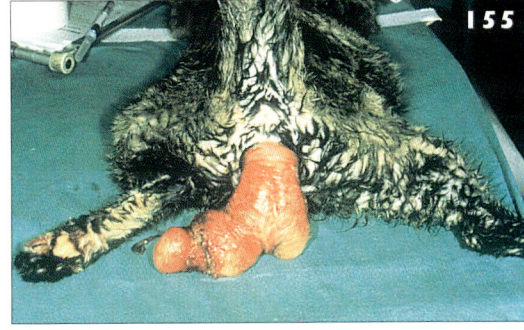

153–155: Answers

153 i. 1.48 liters (0.08 × 18.5). A balanced isotonic, crystalloid solution is a safe choice for this dog.
ii. Hypernatremia results from water loss in excess of solute. Causes of pure water loss: central or nephrogenic diabetes insipidus; possible lack of water intake due to anorexia or withholding of water; hypothalamic dysfunction resulting in decreased thirst; osmoreceptor defect.
iii. $0.6 \times 17.5 \text{ [body weight]} \times (1 - \frac{169 \text{ [desired sodium]}}{190 \text{ [serum sodium]}}) = 1.16 \text{ liters}.$

This volume roughly represents the 1.0 kg (1 liter) weight loss. 5% dextrose in water can be given once the fluid deficit has been corrected. Further correction to 154 mEq/l, with a balanced isotonic solution, can be administered over 24 hours. Chronic hypernatremia should be corrected slowly (12 mmol/kg/24 hours) to avoid central pontine myelinolysis.

154 i. Unless chronic heart failure undetected by the owner is suspected, then an acute onset heart failure would be possible, e.g. ruptured chordae tendinae, possibly subclinical bacterial endocarditis. Otherwise, congested heart failure due to decompensated heart disease, chronic mitral valvular endocardiosis being the most probable cause. Other possibilities include a right to left shunt (Eisenmenger's syndrome) from an undiagnosed congenital defect, though less likely at this age.
ii. Oxygen, furosemide (i/v), topical nitroglycerin and possibly morphine. Echocardiography will evaluate contractility and detect the presence of pericardial fluid. Once the patient is more stable, hydralazine or an ACE inhibitor (e.g. enalapril) is administered orally. If the patient responds poorly, i/v nitroprusside (potent veno- and arteriolar dilator) may be beneficial once an i/v catheter is placed.
iii. Perihilar infiltrates and a mild diffuse interstitial infiltrate is present in the lungs. Pulmonary vessels are mild to moderately enlarged. The cardiac silhouette appears to be at the upper limits of normal. Acute congestive heart failure secondary to ruptured chordae tendinae is still suspected, though bacterial endocarditis of the mitral valve cannot be completely ruled out. An echocardiogram is carried out to assess contractility.
iv. With acute mitral regurgitation, left atrial size is normal and cannot accommodate the increase in volume in acute mitral regurgitation; thus, acute elevation of left atrial pressure produces significant pulmonary congestion. On physical examination the severity of the murmur without previous clinical symptoms and the normal sinus rhythm suggest an acute condition.

155 i. Prolapsed uterus.
ii. The cat should be anesthetized and reduction attempted with lubrication, external pressure and flushing sterile saline into the uterine horns. In this case, external reduction would be unlikely because of the extreme tissue edema and trauma. Ovariohysterectomy is recommended with amputation of the external segment if there is uterine engorgement and necrosis.
iii. Rupture of an ovarian or uterine artery resulting in hemorrhagic shock. Blood transfusion and pelvic counterpressure may be necessary to stabilize the patient before exploratory laparotomy to locate the bleeder and remove the ovaries and uterus.

156 & 157: Questions

156 A four-year-old, female mixed-breed dog is presented after the owners found her outside having difficulty breathing. There is a 1.5 inch (4 cm) skin laceration over the right side of the thorax. The dog has a RR of 80 bpm, with shallow chest excursions. Her head and neck are extended and she appears to be 'air hungry'. Auscultation reveals decreased lung sounds and normal to decreased heart sounds on the right side.

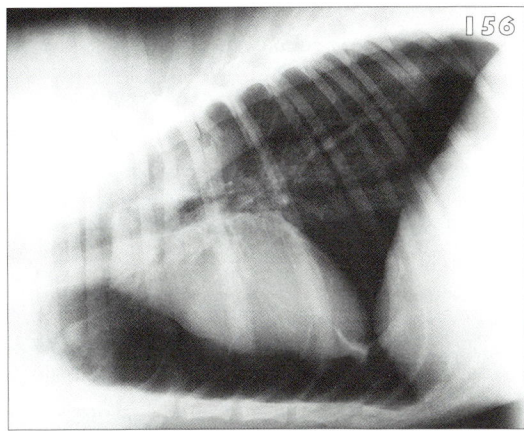

i. What are the differential diagnoses for this presentation?
ii. What is your first course of action?
iii. Radiographs are taken 10 minutes after your initial intervention (**156**). What is your diagnosis?
iv. How would you treat this condition?
v. Although your therapeutic intervention was initially successful, the dog becomes dyspneic again after 30 minutes. What further therapeutic measures should you consider?

157 An eight-year-old, castrated male, orange and white (6 kg) cat is presented with severe depression, vomiting yellow liquid 12 times in the last day, and severe mucoid diarrhea (**157**). The cat had chewed on a lamb chop bone the day before. The cat has a systolic peripheral blood pressure of 60 mmHg (8.0 kPa) with a rectal temperature of 97.9°F (36.6°C). HR is 160 bpm. Dehydration is estimated at 8%. The

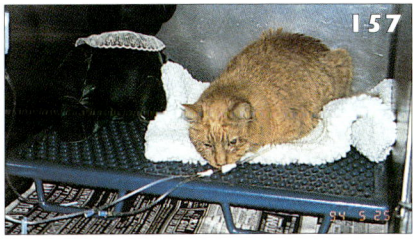

working diagnosis is pancreatitis, a systemic inflammatory response syndrome (SIRS).
i. What three forms of shock are present in SIRS patients?
ii. With this significant hypotension, what major organ is in immediate jeopardy?
iii. In the SIRS patient, what changes are occurring in the small blood vessels, and how can the degree of these changes be estimated?
iv. What is the first and most important therapy for hypotension? How would this be done in this patient, and how would the success be monitored?
v. The most important therapy (see **iv**) has been given and the desired end-point has been reached, except that the cat is still hypotensive (systolic blood pressure – 70 mmHg [9.3 kPa]). What is the next therapeutic step?
vi. The second therapy has been given and the desired end-points of treatment reached. However, the cat is still somewhat hyotensive (systolic blood pressure – 80 mmHg [10.6 kPa]). What is the next therapeutic step?

156 & 157: Answers

156 i. A pleural space disorder (pneumothorax, pleural effusion, diaphragmatic hernia) or severe pulmonary contusions.
ii. Oxygen supplementation, followed by thoracocentesis. If the dog is anxious, and not in shock, sedation should be considered. Radiographs should be taken when the dog is stable.
iii. Pneumothorax with rib fractures.
iv. Therapeutic thoracocentesis. Oxygen supplementation with sedation and/or analgesia, and exploration of the wound to determine if it penetrates the thoracic wall.
v. If thoracocentesis does not restore negative pressure, or if more than three thoracocentesis evacuations do not relieve the pneumothorax, tube thoracostomy with continuous suction should be considered. If the wound penetrates the thoracic wall, a thoracotomy should be considered to allow lavage and exploration of the thoracic cavity.

157 i. Hypovolemic, distributive and cardiogenic shock.
ii. Kidneys.
iii. The vessels are dilated and leaking. The degree can be estimated by looking at the albumin level. If the animal is not losing albumin in the urine and does not have malabsorption or liver failure, the loss of albumin is through the holes in the vessels. This indicates that the holes are big enough for a 69,000 Dalton molecule to pass through. Smaller molecules such as ATIII are likely to pass through. The degree of hypotension and the quantity and type of fluids required to elevate the pressure will suggest the degree of vasodilation.
iv. Ensuring that there is an adequate central volume is the first and most important therapy for hypotension. Fluid resuscitation utilizing a combination of crystalloids and the colloid, hetastarch, should be initiated. Hetastarch should be given at 5 ml/kg increments (given over 10 minutes each time) until the blood pressure is above 80 mmHg (10.6 kPa) systolic and the CVP is 6–8 cm H_2O (3.8–5.1 kPa). Crystalloids are administered concurrently giving an initial bolus of 60–100 ml and then slowed to 35 ml/hour. A CRI of hetastarch is utilized to maintain the colloidal oncotic pressure after the initial bolus resuscitation.
v. Since poor contractility and left ventricular dilatation are part of the SIRS syndrome, the next therapeutic step in this cat would be to give a positive inotrope. Dobutamine (2.5 µg/kg/min CRI) should be initiated. It is ideal to do an echocardiogram to measure chamber sizes and contractility before and after the dobutamine to determine if the desired effects had been obtained.
vi. A vasopressor can be administered. The initial choice is dopamine (5 µg/kg/min CRI). This has mild vasoconstricting effects. The dosage can be adjusted up as needed for the desired results. Care is taken to give the least amount possible for the shortest time since vasopressors can decrease renal and other vital organ blood flow.

158 & 159: Questions

158 A five-year-old, spayed female mixed-breed dog is presented with an acute onset of vomiting yellow foam. There is no history of systemic illness. No medications have been administered. The owner reports that toxin ingestion and trauma are unlikely. Physical examination findings include tachycardia, hyperemic mucous membranes, rapid CRT, bounding femoral pulses and a tense abdomen. Rectal temperature is 103°F (39.4°C).
i. What piece of historical information would you next elicit from this client? (Select one correct answer.)
a. Travel history.
b. Access to garbage or fatty foods.
c. Health of other pets in household.
d. Vaccination status.
ii. What is the most likely explanation for the tachycardia, hyperemic mucous membranes, rapid CRT and bounding femoral pulses? (Select the one correct answer.)
a. Pain and excitement.
b. Fever.
c. Early stage of hypovolemic and/or distributive shock.
d. All of the above.
iii. Your initial lab work and radiographs are consistent with pancreatitis. What treatment will you institute? (Select one correct answer.)
a. Send the dog home on a bland diet and recheck in 2–3 days.
b. Send the dog home with nothing *per os* for 12 hours followed by feeding normal diet.
c. Hospitalize the dog for close observation and give s/c crystalloids.
d. Hospitalize the dog to administer i/v crystalloids and possibly colloids, giving nothing *per os*.
iv. Eighteen hours after beginning fluids the dog appears depressed and is more painful, has not urinated and has petechial hemorrhages on its oral mucous membranes. There is also bloody diarrhea. Assuming that the diagnosis of pancreatitis is correct, what is the most likely explanation for the worsening condition of this dog?
v. How would you treat this patient?
vi. How would you monitor this patient?
vii. Approximately 30 hours after initial presentation, the dog develops sudden onset of respiratory distress and cyanosis. Chest radiographs are basically normal with a questionable hyperlucent area of the right caudal lung lobe. Arterial blood gas analysis indicates hypoxemia, hypocarbia and mild metabolic acidemia. What is the most likely cause of the change in respiratory status? (Select one correct answer.)
a. Pulmonary thromboembolism.
b. Aspiration pneumonia.
c. Pneumothorax.
d. Congestive heart failure.
e. Acute respiratory distress syndrome.

159 A dog was accidentally locked in a walk-in cooler for 1 hour. When found the dog was unresponsive, had a temperature of 89.6°F (32°C) and had shallow breathing.
i. What is the result of hypothermia on metabolism?
ii. What can be the effect of aggressive surface rewarming?
iii. How should frostbite be treated initially?

158 & 159: Answers

158 i. b.
ii. d.
iii. d.
iv. The dog is most likely progressing to the hemorrhagic/necrotic form of pancreatitis. This is a systemic inflammatory response sydnrome and complications include shock, multiple organ dysfunction, DIC and sepsis. The depression and lack of urine production may suggest poor perfusion. The petechial hemorrhages are compatible with low platelet numbers or poor platelet function. The bloody diarrhea may be from GI ulceration or coagulopathy.
v. A combination of crystalloids and colloids would be benefical. Oxygen supplementation would be indicated. Further definition of the potential coagulation problem would be necessary. If there is a declining trend in platelet numbers and a trend for an increasing ACT time, then treatment with heparin and plasma is warranted. Broad-spectrum antibiotics effective against Gram-negative and Gram-positive aerobes and against anaerobes is indicated. Nasogastric intubation for suctioning would help eliminate vomiting.
vi. Monitoring of this patient would include blood parameters such as PCV/TS, glucose, electrolytes and arterial blood gas. CVP and BP assist in determining perfusion status and response to fluid therapy. Urine production should be measured on an hourly basis to see if the aggressive fluid resuscitation has increased urine output. An albumin level should be run to determine the availability of this important intravascular carrier molecule and to give an estimation of the size of the hole in the leaking vessels (if albumin leaks, the hole is at least 69,000 Daltons in diameter).
vii. a.

159 i. Hypothermia causes progressive depression of metabolism, thus decreasing oxygen demand. Oxygen delivery is also reduced through lowered cardiac output, hypoventilation and reduced oxygen transport and delivery.
ii. Surface rewarming induces peripheral vasodilation. As the cardiac output is still reduced, this may worsen the hypotension and induce further hypovolemic shock. Active core rewarming techniques, such as warm i/v and intra-abdominal fluids, lessen the potential of vascular collapse. Whole body rewarming should be gradual, approximately 1°C/hour.
iii. At present it is generally accepted that rapid rewarming of the involved area is the best way to resuscitate the animal. For this purpose the involved area should be placed in water at a temperature of 107.5–111.2°F (42–44°C).

160–162: Questions

160 A 14-year-old cat presented with a sudden total loss of sight and an obvious hyphema completely filling the left anterior chamber. There was no ocular pain and the right pupil remained dilated and non-responsive. Fundoscopic examination of the left eye was not possible but the right fundus is shown (**160**).
i. What is your evaluation of the right fundus?
ii. What is the differential diagnosis for these changes?
iii. What further diagnostics and therapeutics are recommended?

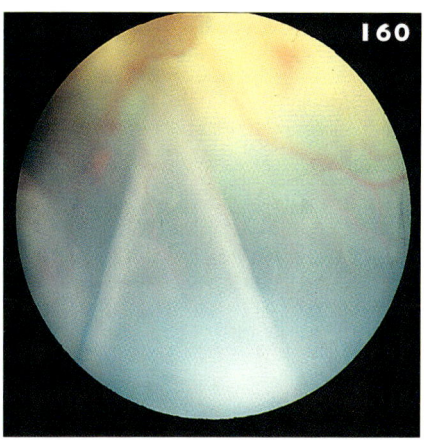

161 A two-year-old, male Dalmatian presents for urethral obstruction (**161**). He is prepared for sedation and unblocking. Multiple attempts at unblocking the ureter with conventional lavage are unsuccessful.
i. What are the options at this point?
ii. If a cystotomy is performed, what intraoperative diagnostic procedures should be performed on the bladder?
iii. What is the most important aspect to performing a urethrostomy?

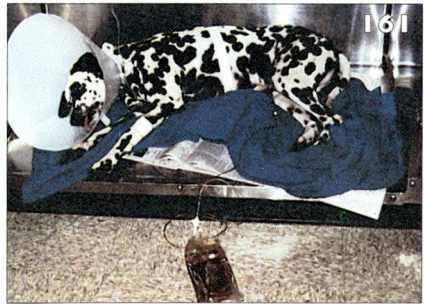

162 A three-year-old, intact female Doberman Pinscher is presented 1 week post-parturient for a vaginal hemorrhagic discharge. Whelping was normal and the puppies are doing well. The dog had been anorexic and depressed for 3 days. An enlarged, fluid-filled uterus is found on abdominal palpation. Rectal temperature is 104°F (40.2°C). The dog is in the compensatory stage of shock. Blood is drawn for CBC and chemistry profile and a large hematoma forms over the vein. The catheter site is bleeding 15 minutes later.
i. Define DIC.
ii. Name three pathophysiologic abnormalities that predispose a patient to DIC.
iii. Describe what is expected to change in coagulation tests very early as DIC is being initiated and how these test results change as the intensity of DIC progresses.
  The coagulation results from this dog were: PT – 13 seconds (normal 8.1–10.1 seconds); PTT – 13.8 seconds (normal 8.1–12.5 seconds); ACT – 130 seconds (normal 90–120 seconds); platelet count – 66,000/mm^3; buccal bleeding time – 6 minutes (normal <4 minutes); FDPs – 10–40 µg/ml (normal <10 µg/ml); fibrinogen – 321 mg/dl (normal 61–178 mg/dl); ATIII – 68% (normal >95%).
iv. Assess the coagulation profile for this dog.
v. Give a treatment plan for this dog related to her coagulation abnormalities.

160–162: Answers

160 i. The right retina is detached and some retinal hemorrhage can be seen.
ii. Bilateral chorioretinitis is a possible differential diagnosis, but it is most likely that secondary hypertension is the cause of the retinal detachment.
iii. Routine biochemistry is necessary to determine the etiology, for it is likely that the hypertension is secondary to chronic interstitial nephritis.

161 i. a. Complete anesthesia ± muscle paralysis while attempting to retrograde flush the obstruction. **b.** Cystotomy and attempts at retrograde flushing. **c.** Prescrotal urethrostomy ± cystotomy and retrograde flushing. **d.** Scrotal urethrostomy ± cystotomy and retrograde flushing. **e.** Temporary cystostomy with a Foley catheter. **f.** Cystocentesis until surgery can be performed (only in extreme emergencies).
ii. Biopsy and culture of the bladder mucosa, and stone analysis and culture of the middle of the calculi.
iii. Suturing the urethral mucosa to the skin to prevent subcutaneous leakage of urine.

162 i. Disseminated intravascular coagulation. This syndrome describes a hypercoagulable state that leads to microthrombosis in the early stages and hemorrhage in the later stages when the coagulation proteins are consumed.
ii. Exposure of blood to subendothelial collagen; exposure of blood to red blood cell phospholipids; release of tissue thromboplastin into the blood.
iii. The platelet count decreases very early in the process of DIC, and ACT may shorten as the patient becomes hypercoagulable. The ATIII decreases slightly from consumption. As the clotting progresses, the fibrinogen begins to decline and the FDPs increase, the amount of increase dependent upon the liver's ability to clear them. The ATIII declines more. As the coagulation factors become consumed, PT and PTT become prolonged, and ACT is prolonged. The platelet count, fibrinogen and ATIII continue to decline and large platelets may become apparent in the blood smear. Overt bleeding becomes evident. The buccal bleeding time may remain normal, depending upon the degree of thrombocytopenia.
iv. The PT is significantly prolonged while the PTT and ACT are mildly increased. This implies that the coagulation factors are beginning to be consumed, with the PT having the fewest factors with the shortest half-life being prolonged first. The platelet count and ATIII are low, implying consumption. The FDPs are elevated, indicating that a hypercoagulable state has occurred and fibrinolysis is ongoing. The fibrinogen may be a reflection of increased production secondary to inflammation, and might possibly be higher if the fibrinogen was not being consumed. The buccal bleeding time elevation can be related to low platelet numbers, but the dog is a Doberman Pinscher and von Willebrand's disease (VWD) must be anticipated until proven otherwise. Impression: DIC with possible VWD.
v. There are five important aspects to treating these coagulation disorders:
• Improve capillary flow and promote tissue oxygen consumption. Aggressive fluid therapy and treatment of hypotension is mandatory.
• Treat the underlying disease. In this case the uterine abnormality must be addressed when the patient is stable enough.
• Support the target organs of thrombosis and hemorrhage. These are classically the heart, lungs, brain and mesentery.
• Provide coagulation proteins and ATIII. This is done through fresh whole blood, stored whole blood, cryoprecipitates or fresh frozen plasma. The selection is made based upon what the animal needs: RBCs?, albumin?, factors V and VIII?, platelets?
• Activate the ATIII with heparin. If the ATIII blood level is adequate, heparin can be given alone. If the ATIII blood level is low, heparin plus the blood products are required.

163 & 164: Questions

163 i. The purpose of a triage system is to:
a. Obtain complete medical history and determine if a patient can be referred to another non-emergency practice.
b. Obtain a complete medical history and obtain TPR, weight.
c. Screen patients into categories based on the severity of illness, and determine their relative priority for treatment.
ii. Following triage, primary and secondary surveys are performed. Which of the following best defines each one of these concepts:
a. Assess and initiate management of life-threatening conditions.
b. Reassessment of vital signs, and rapid, thorough examination of the entire patient from head to tail.
iii. Based on the clinical findings, determine if the patient is the compensatory stage (false stability), middle stage or decompensatory stage of shock:
a. Cyanotic, ashen, white mucous membranes, cold skin, decreased rectal temperature, absent or weak femoral pulses, oliguric, prolonged or absent CRT, losing consciousness, had a seizure.
b. Pale mucous membranes, cool skin, low rectal temperature, weak but palpable femoral pulses, tachycardia, prolonged CRT, mentation (depressed).
c. Normal respiration, red mucous membranes, normal skin and rectal temperature, normal or bounding pulses, tachycardia, normal urine output, CRT <1 second. Mentally alert/conscious (aware of surroundings, mildly depressed to excited).
iv. Knowledge of which conditions cause changes in mucous membrane color is a valuable clinical nursing tool that serves as a diagnostic indicator. Pair each of the following colors to their respective interpretation and cause:

Color interpretation	Causes
Pink	a. Coagulation disorder: platelet disorder, DIC.
Pale	b. Methemoglobinemia: acetaminophen toxicity.
Blue	c. Bilirubin accumulation; hepatic/biliary disorder.
Brick red	d. Hyperdynamic perfusion, vasodilation: early shock, sepsis, fever.
Icteric	e. Cyanosis, inadequate oxygenation: respiratory failure.
Brown	f. Decreased hemoglobin, poor perfusion, vasoconstriction: anemia, shock, epinephrine-induced.
Petechiae/ecchymosis	g. Normal: adequate perfusion and oxygenation at the periphery

164 A five-year-old, spayed female Rottweiler is presented on a hot summer day for weakness, lethargy and ataxia. The dog has been chained without shade in the back yard. Physical examination findings: fever (temperature – 108°F [42.2°C]); tachycardia (HR – 180 bpm); tachypnea (RR – 40 bpm); loud, labored breathing primarily on inspiration; hyperemia of the mucous membranes (CRT – 1 second); and altered mentation. The dog is estimated to be 10% dehydrated.
i. What is your differential diagnosis for this dog?
ii. What are your immediate concerns?
iii. What is your initial treatment plan for this dog?
iv. What further treatment and monitoring would you consider?
v. How would you educate the owners with regard to prevention and first aid?

163 & 164: Answers

163 i. c.
ii. a. Primary survey. Airway maintenance; breathing; circulation; neurologic deficit assessment.
b. Secondary survey. The chest, abdomen, pelvis and extremities are visually inspected, palpated and auscultated where appropriate. Neurologic status is assessed repeatedly.
iii. a – decompensatory stage of shock; b – middle stage of shock; c – compensatory stage of shock (false stability).
iv. Pink – g; pale – f; blue – e; brick red – d; icteric – c; brown – b; petechiae/ecchymosis – a.

164 i. Should include heat stroke, infectious diseases, cardiopulmonary or upper airway disease, seizure activity, poisoning.
ii. Hyperthermia can cause denaturation of cellular proteins, leading to cell necrosis and death. Tissue hypoxia occurs due to increased metabolic demands and poor perfusion. Decompensation of critical tissues such as the brain and heart can lead to rapid deterioration of cardiovascular and neurologic function. Ischemia of the abdominal organs due to shock and hyperthermia can lead to bacterial translocation and sepsis, as well as acute renal failure. DIC and multiple organ dysfunction syndrome are a common complication of this SIRS disease. This is the ultimate SIRS patient, with hypovolemic shock, cardiogenic shock and distributive shock (vasodilation and increased capillary permeability).
iii. The intravascular volume should be rapidly expanded utilizing large molecular weight colloids such as hetastarch, and the interstitial volume replaced with crystalloids such as lactated Ringer's solution. Oxygen should be rapidly supplemented by flow-by methods. Once rapid and aggressive volume restoration is initiated, aggressive cooling techniques are employed (cool water enemas, cool water peritoneal lavage, cool fluids, hosing down with tepid water). Broad-spectrum antibiotics effective against Gram-positive and Gram-negative aerobes and anaerobes are given i/v. Glucose levels are monitored and supplemented as necessary.
iv. Cardiovascular, respiratory, nervous, coagulation and urinary systems are monitored and treated as required. Ventricular tachycardia or VPCs may require lidocaine therapy in addition to oxygen and fluid support. The ECG, BP and CVP should be monitored. The respiratory system is monitored utilizing pulse oximetry, blood gas analysis and end-tidal CO_2. Oxygen is supplemented and ventilation provided as indicated by blood gases or increased respiratory effort. A tracheotomy may be necessary if there is significant laryngeal edema or paralysis. Oliguria is treated with increased renal perfusion and, once rehydrated, a combination of mannitol, furosemide and dopamine at renal doses. The BUN, creatinine and urine output are monitored. DIC is anticipated and heparin is given subcutaneously if the ATIII levels are above 70%. If the ATIII level is lower, then plasma and heparin are administered. The PT, PTT, platelet count, fibrinogen, FDPs and ATIII levels are monitored to assess the status of coagulation. GI hemorrhage is treated with cool water lavage, sucralfate and possibly H_2 blockers. Careful monitoring of serum albumin levels are required to direct plasma infusion to maintain the albumin above 2.0 g/dl. Body temperature is monitored frequently, anticipating a rebound hypothermia following aggressive cooling.
v. Owners should never leave an animal in a vehicle with closed windows and poor air circulation. Outdoor dogs must have shade and access to fresh water at all times. A child's small wading pool is an excellent reservoir of water for large dogs. In case of heat stroke, owners can be instructed to wet the animal's body with tepid water before presentation. Antipyretic drugs such as aspirin or acetaminophen must not be given.

165 & 166: Questions

165 A 12-year-old, castrated male domestic longhair cat was presented for acute posterior paraparesis (**165**). The cat cried out 1 hour ago and could have fallen from a chair. Physical examination found the cat to have paresis of both hindlimbs with painful muscles. There was no pulse in the right hindlimb and a weak femoral pulse in the left hindlimb. Both paws were cold. The cat has a mournful repetitive cry. The mucous

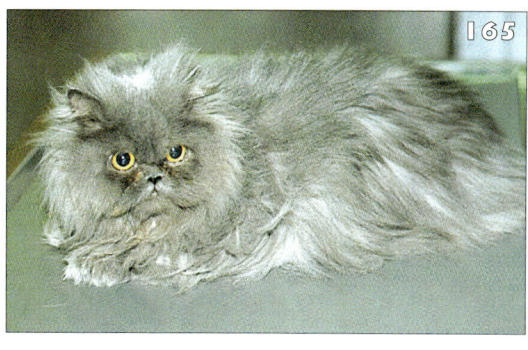

membranes were pale and dry with a prolonged CRT. The heart had a gallop rhythm. Temperature – 96°F (35.5°C); HR – 120 bpm; RR – 25 bpm; PCV – 52%; TS – 8.0 g/dl; BUN by labstick – 50–80 mg/dl; glucose – 160 mg/dl (8.96 mmol/l); Na^+ – 145 mEq/l; K^+ – 7.2 mEq/l.
i. What is your presumptive diagnosis, and with what disease is it most commonly associated?
ii. List other preferred locations for this phenomenon and likely resulting clinical signs.
iii. What is your therapeutic and diagnostic plan for this cat at this time?
iv. What is the prognosis?

166 A ten-year-old, 15 kg, spayed female mixed-breed dog has had significant polyuria and polydipsia for 1 month. Over the last day the dog was locked in a closet by mistake without food or water. The dog presented in lateral recumbency and was stuporous. HR is 200 bpm, the dog is panting, and the mucous membranes are bright red and dry. CRT is 4 seconds. Laboratory results: Na^+ – 182.2 mEq/l; K^+ – 4.86 mEq/l: chloride – 131.5 mEq/l; HCO_3 – 24 mEq/l; plasma osmolality – 357 mOsm/l; urine SG – 1.007; the urine sediment did not have any cells.
i. What is the likely pathophysiology of the CNS signs?
ii. What is the most likely diagnosis of the polyuria and polydipsia described in the history leading to the crisis seen in this dog? How can this be confirmed?
iii. Choose the appropriate fluid therapy (select one):
a. Hetastarch (300 ml) to restore perfusion and lactated Ringer's solution to replace deficit over 12 hours.
b. 0.45% saline (150 ml/hour) to replace deficit over 12 hours.
c. Rapidly infuse 5% dextrose in water (150 ml/hour) to replace deficit over 12 hours.
d. Infuse 0.45% saline (75 ml/hour) to replace deficit over 24 hours.
e. 3% hypertonic saline with hetastarch to restore perfusion and saline to replace deficit over 12 hours.
iv. After perfusion and hydration have been restored, the free water deficit can be replaced. How is the free water deficit calculated?

165 & 166: Answers

165 i. Aortic thromboembolism associated with cardiomyopathy.
ii.

Location	Clinical sign
Brachial artery	Forelimb paresis, pain
Kidney	Azotemia, oliguria, acute renal failure
GI tract	Bowel ischemia, hemorrhagic diarrhea, abdominal pain
Brain	Altered mentation, seizures
Lung	Hypoxemia, respiratory distress

iii. Therapeutic plan: oxygen – flow-by initially and then nasal cannula; i/v catheter; analgesia – butorphanol; furosemide (1–7 mg/kg i/v); nitroglycerin ointment (1/4 inch rubbed into shaved skin of the abdomen); echocardiographic evaluation of the heart for type of cardiomyopathy, medication required and to assess for left atrial thrombus or 'smoke' – if echo evaluation is not available, non-selective angiography can help tell cardiac chamber size and extent of aortic embolism; 2.5% dextrose in 1/2 strength lactated Ringer's solution to provide maintenance and rehydration over 6 hours; BP assessment – if hypotensive, may require colloid resuscitation (5 ml/kg hetastarch), minimize crystalloid infusion if possible; if not hypotensive (or if response to colloid resuscitation) and if no systolic anterior motion of the mitral valve on echo, vasodilator (enalapril at 0.5 mg/kg sid – many authors recommend acepromazine at 0.1–0.2 mg/kg s/c for sedation and vasodilation); treat underlying heart disease (hypertrophic – diltiazem or atenolol; restrictive – digoxin?; dilated – digoxin). Diagnostic plan: repeat BUN after fluids; non-selective contrast study of aorta to determine extent of thromboembolic vessel occlusion (are the kidneys occluded?); radiographs of chest once stable enough. Reported thrombolytic therapy: heparin (220 units/kg i/v followed by s/c dose of 60 units/kg every 6 hours – adjust dose to maintain PT 1.3–1.5 times above normal; streptokinase – i/v loading dose of 90,000 units/cat followed by a CRI of 45,000 units/kg every 12 hours. Heparin is initiated 24 hours after ending streptokinase infusion and during the first several days of warfarin therapy. The cat is maintained on warfarin at home; recombinant t-PA (0.25–1.0 mg/kg/hour i/v for a total dose of 5 mg/kg). Surgical removal of thromboembolus or catheter aspiration of thromboembolism from the artery are aggressive interventions.
iv. Very guarded.

166 i. The hypernatremia causes an increase in plasma osmolality. As the osmolality of the plasma increases, water moves out of the brain cells down the osmotic gradient causing brain cell dehydration.
ii. Diabetes insipidus. Can be confirmed by the administration of aqueous vasopressin.
iii. a.
iv. Water deficit $= 0.4 \times 15 \text{ (lean body weight)} \times \left(\dfrac{182.2 \text{ [serum Na}^+\text{]}}{140} - 1 \right)$

$= 1.8$ liters

167 & 168: Questions

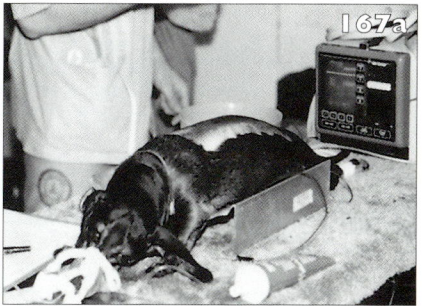
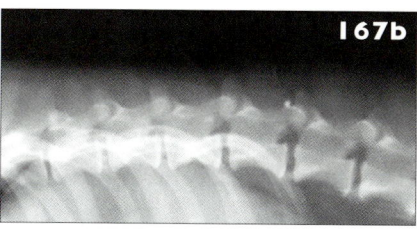

167 A five-year-old, male Dachshund is being prepared for emergency thoracolumbar spinal surgery (**167a**). The owners found the dog dragging its hindlimbs about 4 hours earlier at 5 pm. The dog was noted to walk normally at 12 noon, but seemed wobbly at 2 pm. On your neurologic examination prior to any anesthetic agents, the cranial nerves and forelimbs were normal. There was some voluntary motor movement of both hindlimbs but the dog could not rise on its hindlimbs. A radiograph (**167b**) was taken with the dog under anesthesia.
i. Does this dog have deep pain, and how do you know?
ii. How do you perform a deep pain response test, and what constitutes a positive deep pain response?
iii. Where is the lesion based on this radiograph? (Assume that there are 13 ribs bilaterally.)
iv. List six plain film radiographic signs of acute thoracolumbar disc extrusions. (Do not assume that all of these radiographic signs are present in this case.)
v. What contrast radiographic study is used to localize the surgical lesion definitively?
vi. What are the three potential sources of pain in intervertebral disc disease?
vii. Why is paresis/paralysis less common with acute cervical intervertebral disc disease than with acute thoracolumbar disc disease?
viii. Give two reasons why corticosteroids must be used cautiously in acute intervertebral disc disease.

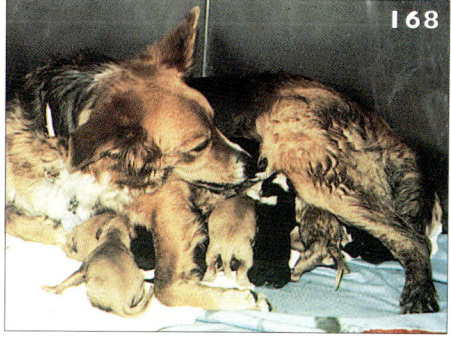

168 This two-year-old mixed-breed bitch finished whelping eight puppies 12 hours ago (**168**). The owner is concerned because the dog has no interest in food, has vomited once, has a dark tarry stool and a copious reddish-brown vaginal discharge, and the body temperature is 103°F (39.4°C). The dog is bright, alert and responsive to the pups.
i. What is your differential diagnosis?
ii. How would you manage this case?
iii. Describe the characteristics of a normal versus abnormal periparturient vaginal discharge.

167 & 168: Answers

167 i. Yes, because deep pain sensation is not lost until after voluntary motor movement is lost.
ii. By applying a noxious stimulus, e.g. hemostats on the toes (to 'crunch bone'). Conscious reaction to the stimulus, such as crying and turning to bite at the stimulus, constitutes a positive deep pain response.
iii. The T12–T13 intervertebral disc space.
iv. Narrowed disc space; small intervertebral foramen; wedging of the disc space; dorsal streaming of disc material from the disc space into the spinal canal; disc material in the spinal canal (cloudiness of the 'horse's head'); narrowing between articular facets.
v. Myelography.
vi. Radicular pain (nerve root impingement); discogenic pain (via pain receptors in the annulus fibrosus and dorsal longitudinal ligament); meningeal pain.
vii. Because there is a smaller ratio of spinal cord diameter to vertebral canal diameter.
viii.
- Corticosteroids can produce euphoria, allowing for 'pain-free' movement by the animal which may potentiate further disc extrusion.
- GI side-effects such as erosions or ulcerations can occur with corticosteroid use. Colonic ulceration has been reported in dogs with intervertebral disc disease treated with corticosteroids.

168 i. Normal post-partum behavior and post-partum endometritis, with the first being the most likely.
ii. The case could be managed in several ways. If the owner wanted to bring the dam to the hospital, radiographs could be taken to ensure that all the pups had been delivered, and cytology performed on the vaginal discharge to rule out a bacterial infection. Oxytocin (5–20 units i/m) could be administered to promote uterine involution and ensure evacuation of uterine contents. If the owner preferred not to bring the dam to the hospital, a house call could be made, or the owner could watch the dog closely and bring her in if she became lethargic and depressed, or if any pups became ill.
iii. The normal lochial discharge indicating placental separation is green to reddish brown and does not have a foul odor. It should not be evident before the first fetus is produced. It normally persists for 2–6 weeks in the bitch and <3 weeks in the queen. The discharge associated with endometritis is purulent and has a foul odor. Cytology reveals large numbers of degenerate neutrophils and intracellular bacteria when infection is present.

169 & 170: Questions

169 An eight-year-old, castrated male Great Dane (75 kg) is presented for retching and non-productive vomiting for the last 4 hours and severe abdominal distension. The dog is triaged as a possible gastric dilatation/volvulus and deemed to be in decompensatory stage of shock. Choose the answer that would be the best approach in each of the patient's treatments.
i. As part of this patient's resuscitation, the nurse should obtain how many venous accesses?

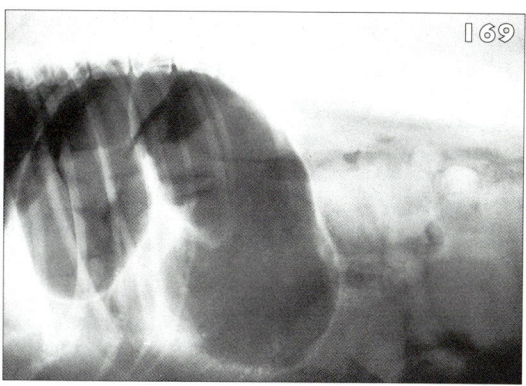

  a. Two 18G i/v catheters, one in each cephalic plus one 18G catheter in the saphenous.
  b. Two 16G i/v catheters, one in each saphenous.
  c. Two 14G i/v catheters, one in each cephalic, plus a jugular central line.
  d. Two 14G i/v catheters, one in each saphenous, plus a jugular central line.
  e. Two 14G i/v catheters, one in each cephalic.

ii. Following decompression the dog develops VPCs. Criteria used to determine if treatment using lidocaine is instituted consist of:
a. More than 10 VPCs/minute with sinus tachycardia.
b. Runs of VPCs, with ventricular tachycardia, poor perfusion.
c. Bradycardia, more than 10 VPCs/minute and pulse deficits.
d. All of the above.
iii. It is decided to give a lidocaine CRI drip at 50 µg/kg/minute. Which of the following options depicts correct steps prior to starting the drip?
a. Start the CRI drip at half dose then increase after 15 minutes.
b. Give an i/v bolus of lidocaine (2 mg/kg), wait 15 minutes and start CRI drip at above rate.
c. Start CRI drip at 75 µg/kg/minute for 15 minutes, then decrease to 50 µg/kg/minute.
d. Give an initial bolus of lidocaine (2 mg/kg). If the arrhythmia converts to normal rhythm but returns to VPCs, give a second bolus at same dose and start the CRI drip at 50 µg/kg/minute immediately.
iv. List four reasons for placing a nasogastric tube following surgery.

170 A dog was shocked by chewing an electrical wire.
i. What is the cause of sudden death in electrical shock?
ii. What type(s) of shock can develop in such a patient?
iii. What types of thermal injuries can be caused by high-intensity currents?
iv. What is a common complication in low-voltage electrical injury in dogs (and cats)?

169 & 170: Answers

169 i. c and e. Because of the gastric distension and the pressure exerted over the blood vessels caudal to the stomach, i/v fluid resuscitation should be given through the cephalic veins. Because of the need to infuse large amounts of fluids rapidly, large diameter short length catheters are used in the cephalics.
ii. b.
iii. d.
iv. Allows nursing personnel continually to decompress the stomach of fluid and air; decreases possibility of regurgitation and aspiration; allows for monitoring of third fluid spacing into the stomach; allows for microenteral nutrition and medication administration.

170 i. When the electrical shock is caused by low voltage (<1000 volts), as in this case, small electrical currents on the myocardium can result in ventricular fibrillation, leading to death. High voltage injury, which is seen infrequently in companion animals, causes cardiac asystole and respiratory arrest, probably due to injury of the medulla of the brain.
ii. Cardiogenic shock results from severe cardiac arrhythmias. Hypovolemic shock develops due to the loss of fluids into damaged tissues and from body surface burns.
iii. Currents passing out of the body surface may generate temperatures as high as 10,000°C and cause extensive carbonification of skin and underlying tissue (arc or flash burns). Such burns often ignite long fur and also cause flame burns. Furthermore, there is injury due to the direct heating of tissues by electrical current through the body. This accounts for tissue destruction greater than expected from observation alone.
iv. Pulmonary edema.

171 & 172: Questions

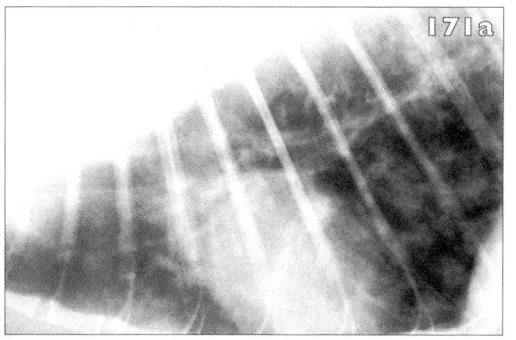
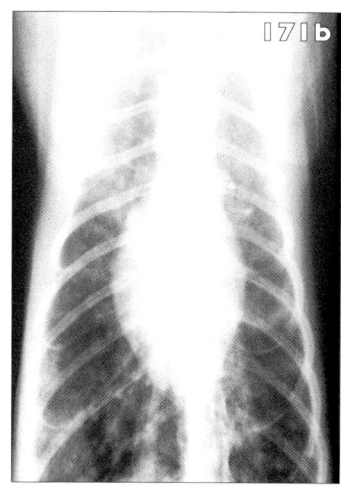

171 A six-year-old, female, spayed domestic shorthair cat was presented with a history of occasional coughing. In the last 12 hours the cat has coughed with increased frequency and is now in significant respiratory distress. Physical examination finds the cat open mouth breathing, 'air hungry' and aggressive. The cat has a prolonged expiratory phase of breathing. Auscultation finds high pitched wheezes and normal HR, rhythm and sounds. The pulses are strong. This is all you can examine.
i. What is your tentative diagnosis from the breathing pattern, auscultation and history?
ii. Describe your initial therapeutic plan and options should the cat worsen.
iii. What radiographic changes do you expect to see?
iv. What are concerns for long-term control?

172 A nine-year-old, entire female Cocker Spaniel presented for vomiting and polyuria/polydipsia of 2 days' duration. On physical examination she was tachycardic (160 bpm), had poor peripheral pulse quality with a blood pressure of 70/40 mmHg (9.3/5.3 kPa), and a prolonged CRT (>3 seconds) with pale pink mucous membranes. She was resuscitated with i/v crystalloids and taken to surgery for an ovariohysterectomy. Postoperatively, a urinary catheter was placed and urinary output monitored.
i. Explain two predisposing factors for acute renal failure in this patient.
ii. Describe the monitoring indicated for renal function in this patient.
iii. Twelve hours postoperatively, this 9 kg patient had a urine output of 2 ml/hour, and her creatinine was 3.8 mg/dl (335.9µmol/l). Following a fluid challenge of 70 ml/hour, her CVP was 8 cmH$_2$O, blood pressure was 115/68 mmHg (15.3/9.0 kPa), and urinary output remained the same. Assuming that the urinary catheter system is functional, what is the diagnosis and what treatment should be initiated?

171 & 172: Answers

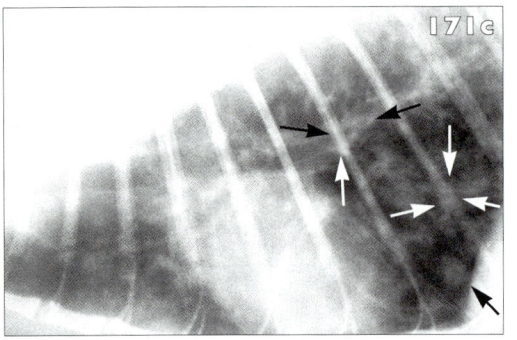
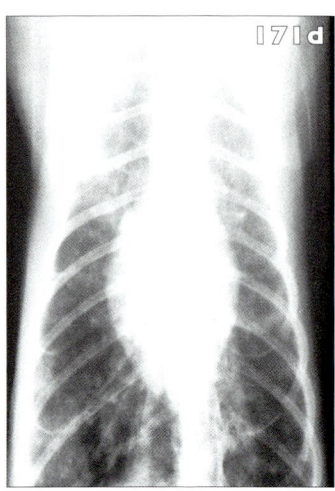

171 i. Feline asthma.
ii. Oxygen by flow-by or small cage; i/v catheter if possible; sedation – butorphanol may be sufficient; fast-acting glucocorticoids; nebulized bronchodilators such as terbutaline (cats will actually seek out this 'mist' and sit with their noses against the outflow spout!).
 Should the cat worsen, epinephrine (1:10,000) (0.25–0.75 ml i/m) can be used, or an albuterol asthma inhaler discharged during an open mouthed inspiration.
iii. Hyperinflation of the lungs; flattening of the diaphragm; bronchiolar markings (**171c**, arrows).
iv. Examination of the environment for inhaled allergens – cigarette smoke is a common initiator. Cats can often be weaned off glucocorticoids and it is then given only as needed by the owner. Should the cat have severe attacks, the owner can keep an albuterol inhaler.

172 i. Hypotension (inadequate for renal perfusion) and sepsis (hypotension, direct toxic damage, microthrombi deposition in the renal vascular bed).
ii. Urinary output (1–2 ml/kg/hour once hydrated and normotensive); urinalysis (checking for renal tubular cell casts, glycosuria in the face of normoglycemia, proteinuria); blood BUN and creatinine; BP (maintain MAP above 60 mmHg [8.0 kPa] for renal perfusion); CVP and PCV/TS for estimation of hydration status.
iii. Oliguric acute renal failure. Initial management requires rehydration and reperfusion. Treatment can be initiated with either mannitol (0.1 g/kg i/v) or dopamine infusion at 1–3 µg/kg/minute with furosemide infusion at 1 mg/kg/hour for 4–6 hours.

173–175: Questions

173 This eight-year-old, female English Setter was referred with continuous vomiting and diarrhea (173). The diarrhea was 'blackberry jam' in color. Physical examination found the dog 10% dehydrated with fluid in the small bowel and no abdominal pain. HR – 180 bpm; CRT – <1 second; mucous membranes – brick red; pulses – bounding. Blood tests found a mature leukocytosis; PCV – 53%; TS – 8.5 g/dl; BUN – 80 mg/dl; creatinine – 4.0 g/dl (353.6 µmol/l); phosphorus – 3.5 mg/dl. Urine analysis: SG – 1.045; negative dipstick; no cells or casts seen on sediment.

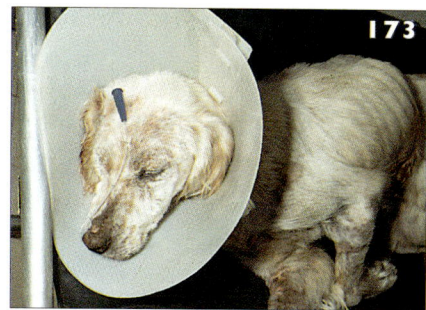

i. What is your assessment of the renal parameters?
ii. What is the initial therapy for this patient?

174 A patient presents with suspected intra-abdominal hemorrhage. A diagnostic peritoneal lavage (DPL) is performed.
i. What is the anatomic site of entry for a DPL?
ii. What position should the dog be placed in, and why?
iii. Why is it important to use a multiholed catheter?
iv. The catheter is placed in the abdomen. What is the next step? What should be monitored?
v. A fluid sample is retrieved from the DPL catheter(174). Based on the PCV on a spun down sample of lavage fluid, when would surgery be recommended?

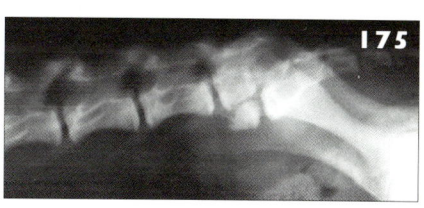

175 An 11-month-old spayed female Labrador Retriever was struck by an automobile about 1 hour prior to presentation. On physical examination, the dog was ambulatory with proprioceptive deficits in both pelvic limbs. Pain was evident upon palpation of the lumbosacral region. A lateral spinal radiograph (175) was taken.
i. Describe the injury on the lateral radiograph.
ii. What part of the nervous system is likely to be injured?
iii. What peripheral nerve reflex is likely to be hyporeflexive?
iv. What peripheral nerve reflex could be hyperreflexive with this injury? Explain how this could happen.
v. Describe how a single stainless steel pin could be used to stabilize this fracture.
vi. What is the prognosis for maintenance of pelvic limb function following repair of this fracture?
vii. What neurologic dysfunction associated with this fracture may worsen the prognosis?
viii. What peripheral nerve is tested by the perineal reflex? From which spinal cord segments does this nerve originate?

173–175: Answers

173 i. The dog has severe dehydration, moderate azotemia and a concentrated SG. The phosphorus and PCV do not suggest any chronicity. The azotemia should be assumed to be prerenal at this time.
ii. Aggressive rehydration and reassessment of renal parameters. Rehydration and reperfusion with crystalloids and colloids improves renal blood flow. Monitoring of CVP will help assess when the venous compartment has been expanded. The underlying disease must be treated.

174 i. 1–3 cm caudal to the umbilicus, modified if palpation indicates a contraindication.
ii. The dog should be in left lateral recumbency which allows the spleen to fall away from the site of entry.
iii. Single holed catheters are more likely to yield negative results.
iv. Infusion of 20 ml/kg warmed isotonic crystalloid solution into the abdomen, stopping if there is any sign of respiratory difficulty.
v. An initial PCV of 20% or more indicates significant intra-abdominal hemorrhage, and surgery should be considered. Surgery should be recommended if the PCV rises >5% above the initial sample after 5–10 minutes.

175 i. The lateral radiograph reveals a cranioventrally displaced L7 spinal fracture.
ii. The cauda equina is likely to be injured.
iii. The sciatic nerve reflex is likely to be hyporeflexive.
iv. The patellar reflex could be hyperreflexive. There are neural communications between flexor and extensor reflex arcs. When the sciatic (flexor) reflex arc is damaged, the loss of flexor inhibition of the femoral (extensor) reflex results in an exaggerated patellar reflex.
v. A transilial pin could be used to stabilize this fracture.
vi. Pelvic limb function is likely to be normal or there may be only proprioceptive deficits.
vii. Injury to sacral nerves may result in urinary and/or fecal incontinence.
viii. The pudendal nerve is tested by the perineal reflex. The pudendal nerve originates from sacral spinal cord segments 1, 2, and 3 (S1, S2, S3).

176 & 177: Questions

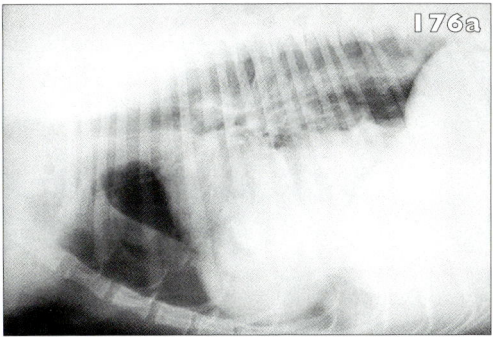

176 A 20 kg, male mixed-breed dog presents after the owner notes the dog has difficulty breathing. He had been treated elsewhere several weeks ago after falling from the back of a truck moving at moderate speed. He has an increase in inspiratory effort with paradoxical abdominal motion. Bowel sounds are auscultated in the chest and there are dull lung sounds in all fields. There is a diaphragmatic rent evident on x-ray, with what appears to be liver, stomach and bowel loops in the thoracic cavity (**176a, 176b**).
i. What are the indications for immediate surgical repair of the diaphragmatic rent?
ii. When is the patient most likely to arrest during the procedure?
iii. Why is it important to prepare the thorax during surgical preparation for abdominal exploration for a diaphragmatic hernia?
iv. Why is it important to prepare the inguinal area and femoral triangle in a critical patient undergoing abdominal surgery?

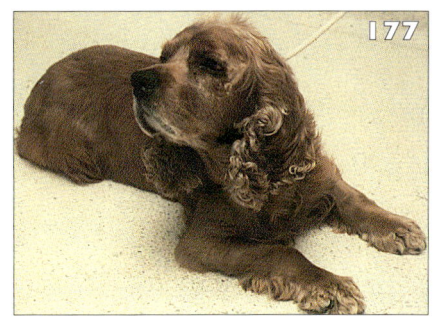

177 A six-year-old, male Cocker Spaniel is referred for evaluation for renal transplantation (**177**). He has been in chronic renal failure for 2 years. The creatinine is now 9.99 mg/dl (884 µmol/l), he is losing weight and is inappetent. The owners would like to know whether the dog is a suitable candidate for renal transplantation.
i. What further work-up on the dog would you require?
ii. What immunosuppressive regimen is currently used in successful long-term, non-matched, canine renal transplantation?
iii. What post-transplant monitoring is essential?

176 & 177: Answers

176 i. Breathing cannot be stabilized medically; abdominal organs are strangulated in the thorax; stomach is in the thorax; shock cannot be stabilized; uncontrolled bleeding in the thorax.
ii. During induction of anesthesia.
iii. There is a potential for lung parenchymal damage that requires examination or resection.
iv. The critical patient may require quick access to the major vessels for instrumentation or large volume replacement. Also, exploration of the caudal abdominal organs may be required.

177 i. Complete physical examination, serum biochemical profile, CBC, urinalysis and culture, chest and abdominal radiographs, and ECG and follow-up of noted abnormalities. Active infection or infection of any form within the past 6 months or neoplasia makes the candidate unacceptable. Chronic, slowly progressive renal failure without infection does not require biopsy (best candidates). Renal biopsy is necessary if the protein:creatinine ratio is >10 (suspect amyloidosis), or if *Borrelia burgdorferi* infection, pyelonephritis without pyuria, or neoplasia is suspected. Renal transplantation is not recommended if vasculitis is present because of the increased risk of thrombosis at the anastomotic site. The personality of the dog is important because of repeated sampling and re-examinations. Owner compliance is essential.
ii. Antidog, antithymocyte serum perioperatively for 7 days; prednisone, azathioprine and cyclosporine in reducing dosage for the lifetime of the patient. However, one of these drugs may be eliminated in time. Newer drugs are becoming available for humans and these may be used in dogs in the future.
iii. Frequent monitoring of urinalysis, urine culture, CBC, creatinine, alanine aminotransferase and whole blood cyclosporine levels are necessary.

178 & 179: Questions

178 A two-year-old Bichon Frise presents with a history of coughing and regurgitating food for several days. He is able to keep liquids down.
i. A radiograph is taken (**178**). What is this, and what are the options for removal?
ii. Other than mechanical obstruction, what is the most common complication of this problem? How urgent is it that the foreign body be removed?
iii. You decide that the foreign body has to be removed surgically. Describe the surgical approach.
iv. What are potential complications of this type of surgery? How may the anatomy of the organ involved lead to complications?
v. How should this patient be fed postoperatively?

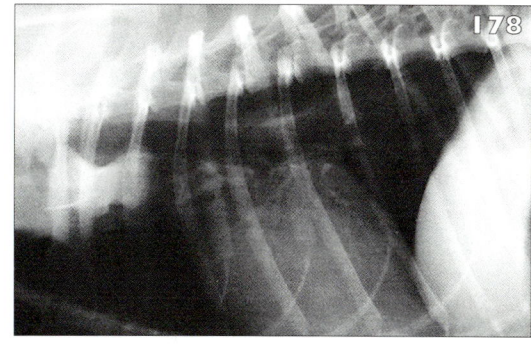

179 A ten-year-old, castrated male dog is presented for weakness and collapse. The mucous membranes are pale pink with multiple small petechiae present. The dog is tachypneic and mildly dyspneic. Lung sounds are normal and multiple areas of petechiation are seen on the abdomen. Only one testicle is present and it palpates normally. Laboratory results: PCV – 22%; TS – 7.2 g/dl; platelets – 25,000/mm^3.
i. Which of the following is NOT an appropriate differential diagnosis for this dog?
a. Estrogen toxicity.
b. Immune-mediated disease.
c. Primary bone marrow disease.
d. Acute whole blood loss.
ii. What is the likely endocrine problem that is causing the problem in this dog?
iii. Does the undescended testicle play a role in this dog's problem?
iv. Blood dyscrasias commonly seen with Sertoli cell tumors:
a. Cause pancytopenia.
b. Result from increased circulating androgens.
c. Cause regenerative anemia.
d. Cause thrombocytopenia.

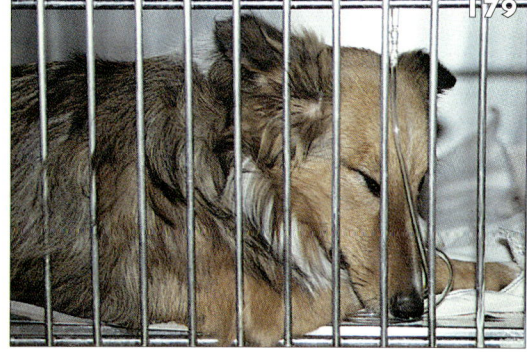

178 & 179: Answers

178 i. Esophageal foreign body. If available, endoscopy (rigid or flexible) is always recommended as the first option. If a flexible scope is being used, it is advisable to use a more rigid tube to dilate the esophagus and then pass the flexible endoscope through it. Extensive lubrication of the tubes and the foreign body with a water soluble jelly will help decrease complications and increase the chance for successful removal. If the foreign body cannot be removed, surgery will be required. On occasion the foreign body cannot be extracted but can be pushed into the stomach and removed via a gastrotomy. This should be done with caution as the esophagus may tear if the foreign body is forced.
ii. The foreign body may cause pressure necrosis leading to pyothorax, pleuritis, pneumonia and possibly pneumothorax. The patient is resuscitated as required to stabilize for anesthesia and the foreign body is removed on an emergency basis.
iii. The thoracic esophagus is most easily approached via a right lateral thoracotomy. The lung is packed off and the affected area of the esophagus exposed. The esophagus is freed up with sharp dissection, being careful to retract the vagus nerve. A longitudinal incision is made in healthy esophagus near or over the foreign body. The foreign body is gently removed. Necrotic tissue is debrided. If a resection is required, esophageal tissue approximately the width of two ribs (placed side by side) can be removed without creating excessive tension during anastomosis. The esophagus is closed in two layers with monofilament suture material. The first layer incorporates the mucosa and submucosa. Pericardium can be used if a patch is required.
iv. Pyothorax can occur secondary to contamination. Wound healing complications may occur due to the lack of a serosa, the lack of omentum and the vascular anatomy. Esophageal strictures may occur when the mucosa and submucosa are extensively damaged.
v. The esophagus should be rested for 3–5 days if surgery was uncomplicated. If a resection or patching were performed, the esophagus should be rested for 7 days. Ideally, a gastrostomy feeding tube is placed at the time of surgery. A feeding tube that comes in contact with the surgical site may cause irritation and should be used with caution; however, small bore soft flexible feeding tubes can be used as a nasogastric or esophagogastric feeding tube. If a feeding tube is not placed, parenteral nutrition should be instituted. Liquids are then initiated and if no problems are noted, the dog is fed a gruel.

179 i. d.
ii. Hyperestrogenism, possibly associated with a Sertoli cell tumor.
iii. Sertoli cell tumors are more common intra-abdominally and seminomas are more commonly seen in the inguinal region, while interstitial cell tumors are not related to cryptorchidism.
iv. a.

180 & 181: Questions

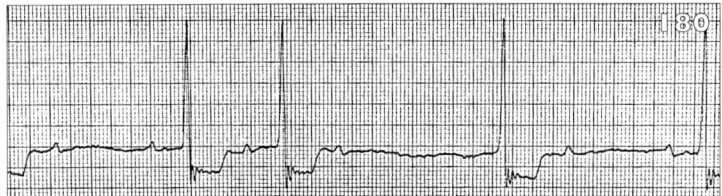

180 A six-year-old, spayed female Doberman Pinscher presents with a 2-day history of anorexia and intermittent vomiting. The owner complains that the dog is extremely lethargic. She has been previously diagnosed with dilated cardiomyopathy and is on furosemide (40 mg bid), enalapril (15 mg sid) and digoxin (0.125 mg bid) in addition to a low salt diet.
i. What is the ECG rhythm diagnosis (**180**), and what does it lead you to suspect?
ii. What diagnostic tests would assist in your diagnosis?
iii. Pending the results of your tests, how would you manage this case?
iv. What are the indications for digoxin? Is digoxin indicated in all cases of congestive heart failure?

181 A six-month-old, female, fully vaccinated German Shepherd Dog-cross is presented with a 10-hour history of 'acting drunk-like and wobbly'. The owner states the dog has 'just slept heavily for the last 3 hours'. After further questioning, the owner informs the clinician that he observed the puppy licking some radiator fluid sometime that morning.
i. The clinician writes orders for i/v catherization and fluids, sedation with diazepam to allow suctioning of the airway, ethylene glycol test, administration of activated charcoal, and taking of blood for potassium, BUN and creatinine estimations. How should the nurse prioritize these orders?
ii. Taking into consideration the estimated time of this dog's exposure (10–12 hours prior to presentation) and the clinical signs with which it presented, choose what two additional in-house tests could aid in the diagnosis of ethylene glycol (EG) toxicosis?
a. Albumin and protein creatinine ratio.
b. Sodium potassium ratio.
c. Serum osmolality and osmolality gap.
d. None of the above.
iii. A urinalysis of an EG toxicosis patient in stage III would most likely reveal:
a. RBCs and triple phosphate crystals.
b. WBCs, RBCs, proteinuria and bacterial rods.
c. Renal tubular epithelial cells, proteinuria (in the absence of RBCs).
d. Calcium oxalate crystals.
e. a and d.
f. c and d.
iv. Ethanol therapy is used as one of the modalities for treating EG toxicosis. Choose the statement that best describes how ethanol affects metabolism of EG.
a. Ethanol binds EG; EG has much greater affinity to ethanol and is thus excreted by the gastrointestinal tract.
b. Ethanol is a competitive inhibitor of alcohol dehydrogenase.
c. Ethanol accelerates breakdown of EG to its metabolites at a faster rate, not allowing time for the accumulation of metabolites to cause toxic effects.

180 & 181: Answers

180 i. First and second degree atrioventricular block. The third QRS complex is a junctional escape beat. Digoxin toxicity is suspected.
ii. Serum digoxin level (toxic >2.5 ng/ml [>3.2 nmol/l]), serum electrolytes (hypokalemia and hypomagnesemia can predispose animals to toxicity even in the presence of 'therapeutic' levels) and a serum biochemical profile (digoxin is eliminated renally; a decrease in glomerular filtration rate results in prolonged elimination).
iii. Conservative measures include discontinuation of digoxin, potassium repletion and appropriate antiarrhythmic therapy. Magnesium administration may be useful in the management of arrhythmias. If there is dehydration and anorexia, begin cautious i/v fluid administration, avoiding overhydration. Restart digoxin at one-half to two-thirds the original dose a minimum of 24 hours after resolution of symptoms.
iv. Two major indications are as a positive inotrope in congestive heart failure and to control supraventricular cardiac arrhythmias (Afib, SVT). Dogs who have evidence of a dilated, failing heart and impaired systolic function may benefit from digoxin. Digoxin is not indicated when congestive heart failure is due to diastolic dysfunction (e.g. HCM).

181 i.
• Suctioning of the pharynx. Because the patient is in stupor, sedation is not indicated. Depressing this patient could add more risk by contributing to the patient's inability to guard its airway.
• I/v catheterization and fluids should be started.
• Blood for ethylene glycol testing should be obtained prior to giving diazepam or charcoal. Drugs such as diazepam and some types of activated charcoal contain propylene glycol or glycerol, which can yield a false positive result.
• No oral medication should be administered unless the medical team has taken control of the patient's airway. Charcoal can be deposited in the stomach via the oro/nasogastric tube.
• Potassium, BUN and creatinine will only serve as base line values unless the patient already has some underlying renal disease, thus placing the patient at higher risk. Stage III of EG toxicosis is acute renal failure and occurs 24–72 hours post-ingestion. Metabolites of EG can chelate calcium and become deposited in soft tissue. Oxalic acid is the primary toxic intermediate, producing tubular epithelial cell necrosis and intratubular obstruction secondary to calcium oxalate deposition. Muscle fasciculation and hyperexcitability often precede toxin related seizures.
ii. c. The EG test is reliable up to 12 hours from the time of ingestion. Serum hyperosmolality and osmolality gap peak at 6 hours post-ingestion and persist for at least 12 hours.
iii. f.
iv. b.

182 & 183: Questions

182 A seven-year-old, male Labrador Retriever (30 kg) is presented with a 1-week history of polyuria, polydipsia, progressive inappetence and recent vomiting (**182**). The dog appears depressed and is estimated to be 8% dehydrated. All palpable lymph nodes are enlarged. Serum chemistry reveals: calcium – 14.96 mg/dl (3.74 mmol/l); creatinine – 2.82 mg/dl (250 µmol/l); albumin – 3.8 g/dl.
i. What is the most likely diagnosis?
ii. What are the differential diagnoses for the hypercalcemia?
iii. What is your treatment plan for the hypercalcemia?
iv. Explain the mechanism by which your treatment plan reduces the serum calcium.

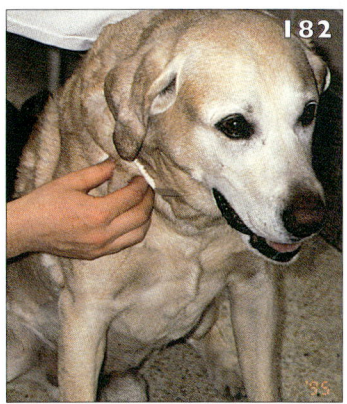

183 A patient is assessed to be bradycardic (**183**) and serum electrolytes reveal a potassium of 10.9 mEq/l. The clinician orders an i/v dose of regular insulin (2 units/kg).
i. What additional precautions should the nurse follow when administering insulin i/v:
a. Give insulin dose followed by fluid bolus and reassess the ECG 15 minutes later. If no change in the ECG, repeat insulin dose at half dose i/v, half dose i/m.
b. Give insulin dose accompanied by 2 g of dextrose per unit of insulin while observing the ECG. The patient is then placed on 2.5% dextrose drip.
c. Give insulin dose and place on 5% dextrose drip. Repeat serum potassium in 2 hours and repeat dose until potassium is less than 5 mmol/l.
d. None of the above. No insulin should be given i/v.
ii. A Foley urinary catheter is placed to monitor urine output. Urine output serves as one of the parameters to assess glomerular filtration rate. Pair the appropriate term to its correlating urinary output:
Normal urine output   a. 1–2 ml/kg/hour
Oliguria   b. < 0.27 ml/kg/hour
Anuria   c. < 0.08 ml/kg/hour
iii. The patient is deemed to be in oliguric renal failure. The clinician writes orders for aggressive fluid therapy and osmotic diuretics. What other two monitoring modalities should the nurse be skilled in and prepared to perform and monitor to assess the patient's response to aggressive fluid therapy?
a. Pulse oximetry and end-tidal CO_2.
b. BUN and creatinine.
c. BP and CVP monitoring.
d. Pulmonary wedge pressure and TCO_2.
iv. CVP is a function of what independent forces:
a. Volume and flow of blood in the vena cava.
b. Dispensability and contractility of the right side heart chambers.
c. Venomotor activity in the vena cava.
d. Intrathoracic pressure.
e. All of the above.
f. a, b and d.

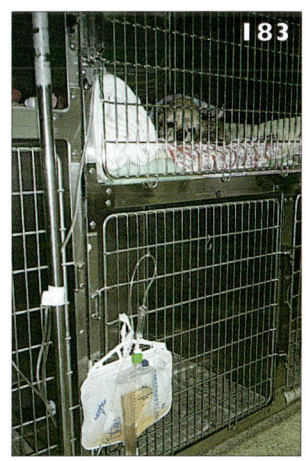

182 & 183: Answers

182 i. Malignant lymphoma.
ii. In descending order of frequency: neoplasia (malignant lymphoma, apocrine gland adenocarcinoma of the anal sac, multiple myeloma, lymphocytic leukemia, metastatic bone tumors, mammary and prostatic gland neoplasia); hypoadrenocorticism; chronic renal failure; primary hyperparathyroidism; hypervitaminosis D (dietary supplement, rodenticides containing cholecalciferol, granulomatous disease); hypervitaminosis A; non-malignant skeletal disease; excessive intestinal phosphate binders. **NB.** Physiologic post-prandial and young animals – laboratory error or lipemia, hemoconcentration, hyperalbuminemia, hypothermia.
iii.
- Correct dehydration: saline is the fluid of choice. Rehydration = $0.8 \times 30 = 2.4$ liters – give half over 6 hours and the remainder over 18 hours. With additional maintenance = 50 ml/hour. Ongoing losses are estimated and added to the hourly rate.
- Enhance renal excretion: furosemide (3 mg/kg i/v) will increase urinary loss. Higher doses (5 mg/kg i/v then 5 mg/kg/hour) have been suggested.
- Treat the underlying disorder. Do not give glucocorticoids until a definitive diagnosis of lymphosarcoma is made or ruled out, unless the hypercalcemia is immediately life-threatening.
- Inhibit accelerated bone resorption. There are several choices: calcitonin (4 units/kg i/v then 4–8 units/kg – effect lasts hours) or diphosphonate etidronate (10–40 mg/kg/day to dogs in divided doses). EDTA (25–75 mg/kg/hour) can be infused. Hemodialysis or peritoneal dialysis with calcium-free dialysate can lower calcium levels. Mithramycin (25 µg/kg once or weekly) is another option.

iv. Volume replacement leads to increased glomerular filtration rate. Saline presents increased sodium and water load to distal renal tubules and calciuresis ensues. As the acidemia is corrected, calcium–protein binding is promoted. Furosemide inhibits calcium resorption in the thick ascending limb of the loop of Henle. Treating the underlying disease reduces the chemical substances responsible for the hypercalcemia. Glucocorticoids reduce the hypercalcemia of lymphoma, multiple myeloma, thymoma, granulomatous disease, hyperadrenocorticism and hypervitaminosis D, with little effect on other causes. Calcitonin and diphosphonates inhibit osteoblastic bone resorption. EDTA combines with calcium and forms soluble complexes which are excreted renally.

183 i. b.
ii. Normal urine output – a.; oliguria – b; anuria – c.
iii. c.
iv. e.

184 & 185: Questions

184 A five-year-old, spayed female Labrador Retriever presented after she was found by the owner having severe grand mal seizures. The dog had previously been healthy and had no history of seizures in the past. The seizures had been occurring over a 90 minute period of time. She presented with a temperature of >106.5°F (41.4°C), tonic/clonic seizures, CRT <1 second, HR of 200 bpm, panting RR and brick red mucous membranes.
i. Along with treatment to halt the seizure activity, what is another major concern in this patient?
ii. What is the initial resuscitation treatment plan?
iii. What complications should be anticipated in this patient?
iv. What parameters should be monitored in this patient?

185 A two-month-old, male kitten is presented with a 5-day history of severe vomiting and diarrhea. The kitten is extremely weak and lethargic. The owner states that the patient 'is so depressed that he has not been able to lift his head for the last 2 days' and last ate 5 days ago. The patient has severe ventroflexion of the neck, bradycardia and 12% dehydration, and is in the decompensatory stage of shock.
i. The team in unsuccessful in establishing a peripheral line. What would be the next method of approach?
a. Give s/c dose of crystalloids.
b. Give oral feeding of oral pediatric electrolyte solution.
c. Perform a jugular cut down.
d. Place an i/o catheter in the femur.
e. Give the fluid i/p.
ii. The patient has a low blood glucose and the clinician orders glucose to be added to 5% in the fluids. The patient has been just started on a liter bag of lactated Ringer's solution. How should the nurse proceed to carry out the order?
a. Spike the liter bag.
b. Use a separate bag to spike with dextrose.
c. Connect to a buretrol and spike only the fluid in the buretrol.
d. All of the above.
e. a and b.
iii. Twelve hours post-resuscitation, serum electrolyte levels are performed and the patient is found to be hypokalemic. What findings on triage assessment are indicative or suggestive of hypokalemia?
iv. On the second day, the kitten is started on kitten growth food gruel every 4 hours. The glucose is now normal and the patient is on a 1% dextrose drip. The nurse notices that 30 minutes post-feeding the patient starts hypersalivating and shows signs of focal twitching. These episodes have been repeated at 4–5 hour intervals. Based on the triage history and present developments, what new differential should be added to the patient's problem list?
a. Juvenile epilepsy.
b. Ingestion of toxins.
c. Hepatic shunt.
d. Insulinoma.

184 & 185: Answers

184 i. The severe hyperthermia and probable hypoxemia.
ii. Therapeutics should include the following:
- Stop seizures with diazepam or pentobarbitol i/v.
- Assure a patent airway and provide oxygen supplementation.
- Volume support with i/v crystalloids and colloids, and supplement glucose as indicated.
- Begin cooling with cool water baths, cool water enemas or peritoneal lavage, and room temperature fluids if temperature is elevated 15 minutes after the seizures stop.
- Broad-spectrum antibiotics against Gram-positive and Gram-negatives aerobes and anaerobes.
- Gastric lavage and activated charcoal if toxicity is possible.
- Head edema protocol (maintain PCO_2 between 35–45 mmHg [4.7–6.0 kPa] and PO_2 at 60 mmHg [8.0 kPa]; keep head flat or slightly elevated to 20 degrees; avoid using jugular vein and keep head position normal; furosemide and mannitol once hydrated and reperfused).
- Nutritional support. The use of glucocorticoids is controversial but has been found to contribute to morbidity in septic patients.

iii. SIRS, DIC, acute renal failure, arrhythmias, shock, impaired cardiac performance, hemolysis, myoglobinuria, hypoglycemia, hypoproteinemia, sepsis, vasculitis, hypoxemia, ARDS, brain edema and swelling, stupor/coma; malnutrition; intestinal sloughing and bacterial translocation.
iv. Perfusion parameters (CRT, mucous membrane color, HR, pulse intensity); urine output and sediment; BP; TPR; CVP; coagulation parameters to include platelet count, ACT or PT and PTT, and ATIII; serial electrolytes; ECG; arterial blood gases; pulse oximetry; end-tidal CO_2. It is very important to follow the Rule of 20 in managing this patient.

185 i. d.
ii. c.
iii. History of profuse vomiting and diarrhea. Ventroflexion of the neck (also seen in thiamine deficiency). Muscle weakness.
iv. c.

186–188: Questions

186 The following question relates to colloid therapy (**186**).
Complete the chart below.

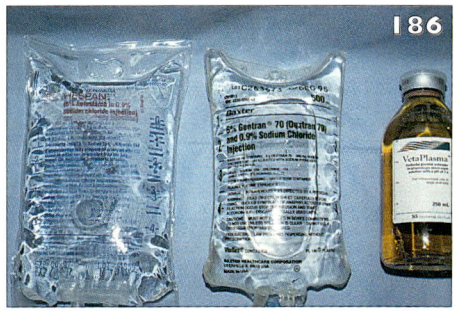

Colloid	Average molecular weight	Half-life	i/v volume increase *
Dextran-40			x 2
Dextran-70		25 hours	
Pentastarch			
Hetastarch	450,000		
Gelatins			
Plasma albumin			

*compared to volume of colloid infused

187 A three-year-old German Shepherd Dog presented with a right forelimb lameness. He had been unobserved for the previous 48 hours. This wound was evident on physical examination (**187**). It was unknown when the injury occurred. The wound was on the medial carpus, involved skin and subcutaneous tissue, and appeared contaminated. Moderate soft tissue swelling and tension was also detected.
i. Is this wound amenable to primary closure?
ii. How could you verify if this wound was infected or not?
iii. Which of the following would not be an appropriate dressing for this wound: biodress; antibiotic ointment and a telfa pad; a wet to dry dressing?
iv. What would you recommend for wound management in this patient?
v. List factors that should be avoided during debridement.

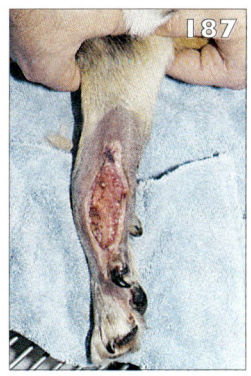

188 An owner calls you concerning an unconscious dog. It is not known why the animal is unconscious: it was normal 2 hours ago.
i. What are your recommendations to the owner concerning transport?
ii. What respiratory parameters do you recommend the owner monitor en route?
iii. If the animal were to stop breathing during transport, how would you advise the owner to proceed?

186–188: Answers

186

Colloid	Average molecular weight	Half-life	i/v volume increase *
Dextran-40	40,000	2.5 hours	x 2
Dextran-70	70,000	25 hours	x 1.4
Pentastarch	264,000	2.5 hours	x 1.5
Hetastarch	450,000	48 hours	x 1.3
Gelatins	35,000	2.5 hours	x 2
Plasma albumin	69,000	16 hours	x 1

*compared to volume of colloid infused

187 i. Infection and tension are contraindications to primary closure of this wound.
ii. Rapid slide test, tissue cultures and biopsy techniques. Wounds that contain >10^5 bacteria/gram of tissue are considered to be infected and should not be closed.
iii. Occlusive dressings such as biodress are not recommended for infected wounds.
iv. This wound should be managed open, because infection is expected. Wet to dry bandages work well. The wound could be left to heal by contraction and epithelialization. If a wound can be converted to a clean wound with debridement and excessive tension is avoided, it may be closed primarily.
v. Prolonged pressure of retractors; excessive grasping of skin edges with tissue or thumb forceps; excessive tension on tissues; massive ligatures with strangulation of tissue distal to the ligature; excessive dissection of tissue planes that can spread infection; excessive electrocoagulation resulting in areas of necrotic tissue.

188 i. Immediate transport to the hospital is advised. The head is kept level with the body or elevated to 20 degrees. The head is in a normal 45 degree angle to the neck. Do not wrap the neck or tape it to a board because struggling can worsen injuries. ICP can rise acutely with jugular vein distension.
ii. Respiratory rate, effort and pattern can be monitored. Non-pigmented gum color can be monitored for abnormal pale, gray or blue coloration.
iii. Mouth to nose ventilation can be initiated. The mouth is closed and 3–4 breaths are delivered quickly into the nostrils. This is followed by 10–12 bpm. The owner can pinch behind the trachea to occlude the esophagus. Chest compressions are initiated when no pulse or heart beat is detected.

189 & 190: Questions

189 i. Assessment of a patient's acid–base status reveals severe metabolic acidosis and hypocalcemia. The patient is receiving lactated Ringer's solution (LRS). The clinician orders supplementation of sodium bicarbonate and calcium. Choose one of the two options within the parentheses that would correctly complete the following statement as to what precaution the nurse should take when carrying out these orders.
a. Sodium bicarbonate should not be added to fluids containing (calcium, potassium). (LRS, Plasma-Lyte A) contains calcium and should not be used. A better choice would be (sodium chloride, LRS).
b. Sodium bicarbonate supplementation is most carefully infused using (buretrol chamber, primary fluid bag) or infusion pump, to ensure proper dosage delivery.
c. Overtreatment with sodium bicarbonate can result in (hyponatremia, hypernatremia), (hyperosmolality, hypo-osmolality), volume overload, (acidosis, alkalosis), paradoxical CSF acidosis, cerebrospinal fluid, (ionized, total) calcium shifts, and seizures.
d. Calcium should not be added to fluids containing sodium bicarbonate, since precipitated (calcium carbonate, calcium lactate) will form. It should not be added to fluids containing phosphates since calcium phosphates will form.
e. Excessive or too rapid infusion of calcium i/v can cause cardiac arrest, preceded by (bradycardia, tachycardia).
f. Calcium supplementation should be given using calcium gluconate, because the effects of (calcium chloride, calcium gluconate) are three times more potent.
ii. The patient is to be started on peritoneal dialysis. Prior to catheter insertion, what data and/or procedures should the nurse carry out? a. Patient's weight and vital signs to establish base line values. b. Have patient void or manually express the urinary bladder. c. Base line CBC, serum chemistries and electrolytes. d. All of the above. e. a and c.
iii. The most common complication of peritoneal dialysisis is peritonitis. The nurse should use aseptic techniques to prevent such complication. Which of the listed precautions or considerations should the nurse follow? a. Wear gloves and wash hands before and after handling patient. b. Cover catheter site with povidone-iodine soaked gauze. c. Cover all peritoneal dialysis junction sites with povidone-iodine soaked gauze. d. Change all connection tubing from dialysis bag to patient every 6 hours. e. Maintain all lines including drainage bag off the floor. f Examine outflow fluid (effluent) for color and clarity; perform microscopic evaluation of fluid once a day.
iv. During peritoneal dialysis for removing substances from the blood, which indwelling time and drain time is best?
a. 45 minute indwelling time, 15 minute draining time.
b. One hour indwelling time, 1 hour draining time.
c. Two hour indwelling time, 1 hour draining time.
d. All the above.

190 A 20 kg male Dalmatian presents after being hit by a car. His gum color is white with a 4 second CRT. HR is 120 bpm; pulses are weak and thready. The dog has a labored inspiration and expiration with an abdominal grunt. There is an open bleeding fracture of the right femur and bilateral epistaxis. The dog is mentally dull.
i. What stage of shock (compensatory, early decompensatory, decompensatory) is this patient in? Justify the selection.
ii. What physiologic mechanism has failed that allows intracellular calcium to build up during tissue hypoxia?
iii. Immediate fluid resuscitation is paramount. However, reinstituting circulation and oxygen flow to ischemic tissues is not without consequences. What are these consequences?

189 & 190: Answers

189 i. a. calcium; lactated Ringer's solution; sodium chloride.
b. buretrol chamber or infusion pump, to ensure proper dosage delivery.
c. hypernatremia, hyperosmolality, alkalosis, ionized.
d. calcium carbonate.
e. bradycardia.
f. calcium chloride.
ii. d.
iii. All except d. Dialysis tubing is changed once every 24 hours. Handling or manipulating lines more often increases the chances of contamination of port and junctions.
iv. a.

190 i. Decompensatory shock. Perfusion is poor as evidenced by the poor membrane color, prolonged CRT and poor pulse quality. The dog's cardiovascular system is not responding appropriately; instead of the heart rate being increased it is decreased. It is possible that the heart and brain are starting to fail.
ii. The sodium-potassium ATPase pump keeps sodium levels in the cytoplasm at a level that cellular swelling does not occur. In addition, it keeps intracellular calcium levels at a minimum so that calcium activated proteases are not produced in excess. This pump and other calcium pumps require energy derived from aerobic metabolism of glucose. When oxygen is not available, calcium builds up within the cytoplasm.
iii. Reperfusion of hypoxic tissue causes calcium activated proteases to catalyze xanthine oxidase in the formation of oxygen radicals. These radicals are directly toxic to the cell membranes, causing lipid peroxidation and induction of the arachidonic acid cascade. Cytokines are released, and a systemic inflammatory response begins.

191 & 192: Questions

191 A ten-year-old, spayed female Dachshund presents with respiratory distress and with a history of a heart murmur for which she is receiving long-term furosemide therapy. On primary survey the patient has a prolonged CRT of 3 seconds, pale gray gum color, a heart rate of 120 bpm and weak femoral pulses. Pulmonary auscultation reveals moist crackles in all fields. There is a 5/6 heart murmur auscultated during systole. The patient is estimated 6% dehydrated based on skin turgor.

i. Fill in the appropriate sections regarding shock:

Type	Initiating Factor	
	CO*	SVR**
Hemorrhagic	Reduced	
Septic		Decreased
Distributive		
Cardiogenic		
Obstructive		

*cardiac output
** systemic vascular resistance

ii. Which types of shock is this dog experiencing?
iii. What choice of fluid therapy is appropriate for this patient?

192 This six-year-old, castrated male Miniature Poodle developed multiple ecchymotic areas (**192**) on the ventral abdomen following the suturing of bite wounds sustained 1 day prior. His owners had reported that following the trauma and suturing of the wounds, the dog had been extremely lethargic for the subsequent 24 hours prior to presentation.

i. What is the likely complication?
ii. Explain the pathogenesis of the complication seen in this patient.
iii. What specific parameters should be monitored which pertain to the observed complication of sepsis in this dog?
iv. Outline the five components of treatment of this complication.
v. Why is the measurement of ATIII important in this patient?

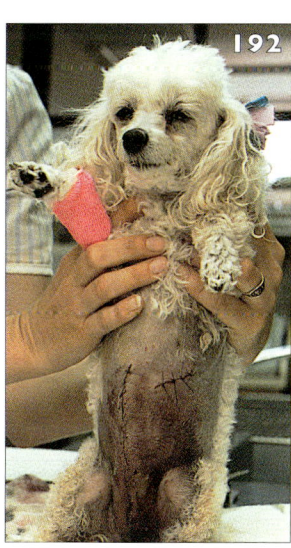

191 & 192: Answers

191 i.

Type	Initiating Factor	
	CO*	SVR**
Hemorrhagic	Reduced	Increased
Septic	Increased	Decreased
Distributive	Reduced	Decreased
Cardiogenic	Reduced	Increased
Obstructive	Normal	Increased

*cardiac output
** systemic vascular resistance

ii. A component of cardiogenic shock, as evidenced by the clinical signs of heart failure and poor perfusion. In addition, there is a component of hypovolemic shock as this dog is on long-term furosemide and appears dehydrated.
iii. Interstitial rehydration with a replacement fluid. Maintenance fluids, such as 2.5% dextrose in half strength lactated Ringer's solution, are appropriate for maintenance of intravascular volume in the heart failure patient.

192 i. DIC due to shock and probable sepsis.
ii. Endothelial and tissue damage secondary to ischemic damage, hypoxia, endotoxin and cytokines expose collagen and thromboplastins to the systemic circulation. Endotoxin and cytokines can also directly initiate the intrinsic coagulation pathways. Tumor necrosis factor, platelet activating factor and thromboxane A2 are three cytokines released during SIRS/sepsis that can separately initiate a hypercoagulable state.
iii. Minimal monitoring would include ACT and platelet estimates. Ideally, PT, APTT, platelet count, fibrinogen levels, FDPs and ATIII levels would help make the diagnosis.
iv.
• I/v fluid administration and BP support to improve perfusion.
• Treat the underlying disease.
• Support target organs which are especially vulnerable to microthrombi damage (lungs, kidneys, brain, intestines, heart).
• Replacement of ATIII and active coagulation factors with transfusion of fresh frozen plasma.
• Heparin therapy to activate ATIII.
v. ATIII values, when decreased, are diagnostic of a hypercoagulable state. A decreased ATIII is one of the earliest known indicators of a hypercoagulable state, which is often caused by DIC. ATIII levels also aid in guiding heparin therapy used for DIC treatment. Since heparin functions by accelerating the reaction of ATIII with thrombin, there is no benefit in administering heparin if there are inadequate levels of ATIII.

193–195: Questions

193 A ten-year-old German Shepherd Dog presents in acute collapse with pale mucous membranes, weak pulses, tachycardia and a marked increase in respiratory effort. Abdominal palpation reveals a cranial abdominal mass effect and a fluid wave (**193**).
i. What is the most likely diagnosis?
ii. What is the best way rapidly to control hemorrhage from the affected organ at surgery?
iii. Care must be taken to ensure that the blood supply to what nearby organ is preserved?
iv. What intra-abdominal organ can be incorporated into the suture to aid with hemostasis?

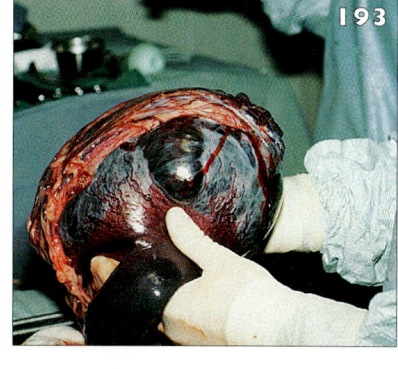

194 A nine-year-old, spayed female Schnauzer presented with a diagnosis of diabetic ketoacidosis 48 hours ago (**194**). Prior treatment was fluid therapy, regular insulin and ampicillin for urinary tract infection. The patient responded well but now has pale gums. PCV is 20% (38% 1 day ago) and the serum is hemolysed.
i. What is the most likely cause for the anemia?
ii. List differential diagnoses for this cause.
iii. What is the mechanism of this cause in this dog?
iv. What other clinical signs may develop from this cause?
v. How would you treat this problem?

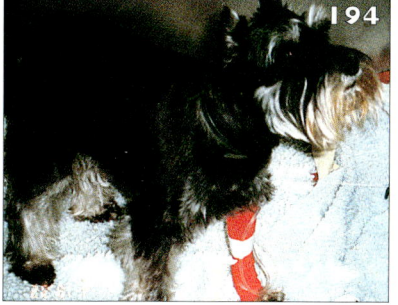

195 An 8-year-old FS Cocker Spaniel presents in fulminant congestive heart failure. She has a grade 3/6 holosystolic murmur heard loudest on the left. Chest films show interstitial and alveolar lung infiltrates in all lung fields that obscure the cardiac silhouette. Echo finds dilated left ventricle and thin walls and septum(**195**). An ECG shows sinus tachycardia at 160 bpm.
i. What is the most likely echo diagnosis?
ii. What would be your immediate therapy at initial presentation?
iii. The dog has a contractility of 12%. What do you do?
vi. How would you manage the afterload in this dog? The dog has been stabilized for 10 hours and is receiving 30 ml/h i/v fluids. He has been weaned from the intravenous afterload reducing agents and is on maintenance oral enalapril. He is also receving i/v furosemide, oral digoxin at a maintenance dose and is being weaned from his positive i/v inotrope. His indirect blood pressure drops over two hours to 70/50 mmHg (9.3/6.7 kPa).
v. What do you do and why?

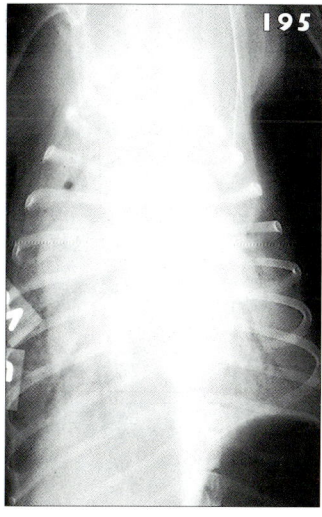

193–195: Answers

193 i. A ruptured spleen – usually hemangiosarcoma in this age and breed of dog.
ii. A vascular clamp or loop should be placed immediately on or around the splenic vascular pedicle.
iii. The pancreas.
iv. The omentum can be sutured onto or around the bleeding area.

194 i. Hypophosphatemia.
ii. Treatment of diabetic ketoacidosis with fluids and insulin (and bicarbonate if administered); re-feeding after prolonged starvation; total parenteral nutrition; transfusion of old stored blood; severe burns; recovery from severe hypothermia; hypomagnesemia; hyperparathyroidism; phosphate binders; renal tubular disorders; respiratory hyperventilation/alkalosis; eclampsia; hypovitaminosis D; cardiac abnormalities; feline hepatic lipidosis; laboratory error.
iii. Patients with diabetes mellitus have a total body deficit of phosphate due to loss of muscle mass, urinary phosphate losses and tissue utilization of phosphate associated with insulin deficiency. It is manifested after rehydration and extracellular to intracellular movement promoted by insulin.
iv. Anemia with hemolysis, muscle weakness and pain from rhabdomyolysis, obtundation, stupor, coma or seizures due to cerebral dysfunction, sepsis due to leukocyte dysfunction, and thrombocytopenia.
v. Serum phosphorus level is <0.4 mEq/l before clinical signs are apparent. Therapy is potassium or sodium phosphate (0.01–0.03 mEq/kg/hour over 4–6 hours). If potassium is administered, make sure it is given at a rate of <0.5 mEq/kg/hour.

195 i. Dilated cardiomyopathy of Cocker Spaniels.
ii. Oxygen, furosemide at 2–7 mg/kg i/v, 0.25 inch (0.5 cm) of nitroglycerine paste applied to the shaved area of skin, possibly narcotic such as morphine for venodilation, sedation, and relief of anxiety.
iii. Begin dobutamine at 5–10 μg/kg/min by CRI and oral digoxin for maintenance therapy at home.
iv. Afterload is reduced with arterial dilating drugs such as angiotensin-converting enzyme inhibitors (e.g. enalopril, benazepril, captopril) orally, hydralazine orally, or nitroprusside or nitroglycerine intravenoulsy by CRI. Mild-to-moderate pulmonary edema is often best managed with oral afterload reducing agents. However, fulminant pulmonary edema may require immediate arterial dilation with nitroprusside. The dose is started at 0.5–1 μg/kg/min CRI and titrated to effect. The optimal end-point of titration is maintenance of arterial blood pressure, lowering heart rate and improved ventilation and oxygenation. Improvement may be evident within 15–20 minutes of finding the right dose. Extreme care must be taken to avoid hypotension. A metabolic by-product of long term nitroprusside administration is cyanide.
v. Check the drug dosages and make sure the arterial dilating agents are at a proper dose. Confirm that contractility has improved, and then consider that the dog may be hypovolemic from diuretic administration. A small fluid challenge may be warranted, using a large molecular weight colloid such as hetastarch at 5 ml/kg, and check for improvement of blood pressure.

196 & 197: Questions

196 A decision is made to perform an exploratory laparotomy due to evidence of significant abdominal hemorrhage (**196**).
i. What are the criteria for making a decision on medical versus surgical management of a bleeding abdomen?
ii. The patient is surgically prepared to include the caudal half of the thorax and the inguinal regions. Why?
iii. Describe the procedure for attempting to control immediately intra-abdominal hemorrhage using digital pressure once the incision is made through the linea alba.
iv. After placing direct pressure on the cranial abdominal aorta, what is the next step?
v. What is the next step after the bleeding areas of the abdomen have been packed?

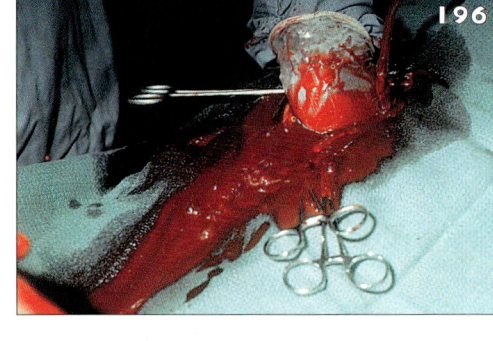

197 i. What are the indications for diagnostic peritoneal lavage (DPL)?
ii. How is a DPL performed?
iii. Match the following five DPL findings with the appropriate interpretation and course of action:

1. Clear fluid; <500 mature neutrophils/mm^3; creatinine – 8.0 mg/dl (707.2 µmol/l) (serum creatinine – 3.5 mg/dl [309.4 µmol/l]); K$^+$ – 10 mEq/l) (serum K$^+$ – 4.5 mEq/l).

2. Fluid slightly turbid; 15,000 neutrophils/mm^3; toxic change in many neutrophils; bacteria present within neutrophils and macrophages.

3. Brown, foul-smelling fluid obtained on insertion of lavage catheter; cytology reveals a mixed population of bacteria, some debris and few **WBC**s.

4. Pink fluid with **PCV** – 20%; cytology reveals many RBCs; peripheral **PCV** – 31%.

5. Slightly turbid fluid; 10,000 mature neutrophils/mm^3; no bacteria seen. Peripheral **WBC** count 22,000/mm^3 with mature neutrophilia and mild left shift. Patient had surgery to remove infected uterus three days prior to lavage.

a. Septic peritonitis – stabilize patient and perform exploratory laporotomy as soon as possible.

b. Mild hemoperitoneum – if patient is stable, repeat lavage and peripheral **PCV** determinations in 1–2 hours. If ongoing hemorrhage is present, consider exploratory laparotomy if coagulation parameters are normal.

c. Punctured bowel loop with catheter with fecal contamination – remove catheter and repeat lavage in different location looking for signs of peritonitis.

d. Uroperitoneum – stabilize patient and proceed to surgery as soon as feasible.

e. Normal in this setting.

196 & 197: Answers

196 i. A hemoabdomen should be explored if abdominal expansion is more clinically apparent and one of the following exists:
• Vital signs (HR, BP) not responding to volume expansion and counterpressure.
• Radiographic signs of pneumoperitoneum, diaphragmatic hernia or mass effect.
• Presence of abdominal herniation or penetration.
• PCV of sample of diagnostic peritoneal lavage fluid taken within 5–10 minutes of initial sample >5% greater than initial sample.
• Microscopic or chemical analysis of fluid suggesting hollow viscus leakage (i.e. intestine, urinary bladder, gallbladder).
• Radiographic or ultrasonographic evidence of continued retroperitoneal space expansion despite use of counterpressure.
ii. The wide area prepared allows the surgeon to perform a parasternotomy/sternotomy in cases of uncontrollable abdominal hemorrhage for possible aortic cross-clamping. It also allows access to femoral veins and arteries for vascular access for fluid administration and direct pressure monitoring.
iii. The incision in the linea alba should be large enough to just allow placement of the hand into the abdomen, advancing along the abdominal wall cranial to left kidney. Move the finger(s) to the midline cranial to the left adrenal gland and apply pressure to the aorta, thus controlling arterial hemorrhage caudal to the cranial mesenteric artery.
iv. The abdomen should be packed with sterile towels, gauze or laparotomy pads, with the aim of placing direct pressure on bleeding areas.
v. All four quadrants of the abdomen are explored one at a time, with immediate control of bleeding.

197 i. Acute abdominal pain; concern for ongoing hemorrhage; fever of unknown origin; known penetrating trauma to the abdomen; known blunt trauma to the abdomen and can not stabilize patient; other history that would support peritonitis from any cause; loss of detail on abdominal radiographs; fluid seen on abdominal ultrasound that could not be aspirated; other.
ii. The abdomen is clipped and aseptically prepared. A large bore over-the-needle or J-wire-guided catheter long enough to be inserted clearly into the abdominal cavity is used. Some drainage holes are made in the sides of the catheter, taking care not to cut the holes too big and making sure that the hole edges are smooth. A small amount of local anesthetic is placed at the entry site (usually just caudal to the umbilicus on the midline). Careful palpation is required to be sure that distended organs or masses are not damaged. It is best if the animal empties its urinary bladder prior to catheter insertion. The abdomen is prepared again and a small skin incision is made with a scalpel blade. The catheter is then inserted into the abdomen in a caudal direction. It is advanced slowly so that any bowel that might be in the way can move. Any fluid that drips freely from the catheter is collected in sterile sample collection tubes. If no fluid is retrieved, 10–20 ml/kg of warm, sterile saline is administered into the peritoneal cavity. The catheter is capped and the dog is allowed to move about and distribute the fluid throughout the abdomen. Then the fluid is withdrawn and saved for biochemical, bacterial and cytologic examination. Do not expect to get much fluid back.
iii. 1 – d; 2 – a; 3 – c; 4 – b; 5 – e.

198 & 199: Questions

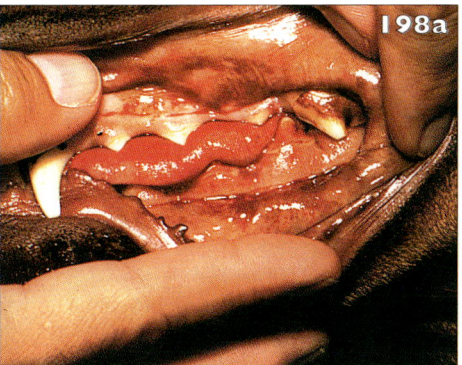
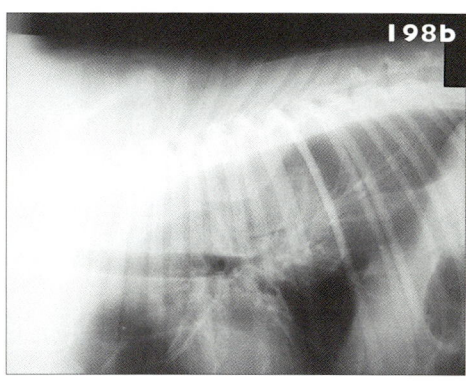

198 An 11-month-old, male Doberman Pinscher is presented with a 3-day history of coughing. In the past few hours he has started to produce frank blood and blood clots when he coughs (**198a, 198b**).
i. Based on the clinical presentation, what historical questions should be asked of the owner?
ii. What diagnostic tests are indicated?
iii. Your initial diagnostic tests reveal an ACT of 3 minutes and a normal platelet estimate. What initial treatment would you implement?

199 A four-year-old Golden Retriever presents shortly after having been hit by a car. The dog is collapsed and showing evidence of moderate respiratory difficulty, with dysynchronous (chopping) movements of the chest and abdomen. Lung sounds are auscultable bilaterally; however, they are very dull on the left side.
i. What is the first line of treatment?
ii. If you suspect intrapulmonic hemorrhage, can the body position of the dog have any effect on the degree of respiratory difficulty the dog is experiencing? If so, how should the dog be positioned?
iii. I/v fluids are started as well. Would your next step be to take a chest radiograph or perform a thoracocentesis?
iv. A thoracentesis is performed and a large amount of blood is retrieved. What criterion is used to determine whether or not to place a chest tube (to treat a hemothorax)?
v. When a patient has a hemothorax, what criteria are used to determine whether the blood should be evacuated or not?
vi. What criteria are used for making a decision to perform an exploratory thoracotomy to control hemorrhage?
vii. What are the likely sites of hemorrhage in a hemothorax?

165

198 & 199: Answers

198 i. Possible exposure to rodenticides, previous bleeding episodes (e.g. following spaying or castration) which might indicate a coagulation factor deficiency, and recent use of medications which could cause platelet function disorders, vitamin K malabsorption or immune-mediated thrombocytopenia.
ii. A coagulation profile is indicated, including a platelet count, PTT, PT and assays for fibrin degradation (or split) products and fibrinogen. An ACT and platelet estimate on a blood smear may help to indicate a coagulopathy. Thoracic radiographs are indicated to determine the source of the hemoptysis.
iii. Rodenticide toxicity is suspected. Treatment should consist of vitamin K1 therapy (loading dose of 5 mg/kg s/c then 2.5–5.0 mg/kg/day p/o), plus supportive care including oxygen supplementation if tachypneic or dyspneic, and whole blood or plasma replacement if indicated.

199 i. High flow oxygen.
ii. If hemorrhage into one lung or one side of the chest is suspected, the injured side should be placed dependent. This may help prevent blood from mixing with air in the healthier lung and can have a major impact on the degree of hypoxia. The upside lung is easier to inflate fully – gravity makes the more dependent areas harder to inflate.
iii. A thoracocentesis should always be performed first.
iv. Evidence of penetration trauma; if there is >20 ml/kg blood evacuated from the thorax; if a thoracocentesis is performed more than twice to evacuate blood; if blood removed on a second thoracocentesis is more than the first thoracocentesis; or if there is a concurrent pneumothorax.
v. If the hemothorax is interfering with ventilation, it should always be evacuated. Current human recommendations for evacuation of a hemothorax include the following:
• Greater than one-third of one hemithorax is blood-filled.
• One lobe is atelectatic because of the hemothorax.
• The hemothorax is associated with a fever spike.
vi. If the patient is 'dying before your eyes' from a thoracic injury, an emergency thoracotomy should be performed. If there is evidence of penetrating trauma or if the patient is not stabilizing with conservative management (chest tubes, oxygen and volume support), an exploratory surgery should always be performed.
vii. Animals that have injuries to the great vessels or the heart usually do not survive long enough to make it to the hospital. The injuries that have the best prognosis are those that are in a low pressure system such as the pulmonary arteries and veins. Intercostal vessels when transected can cause severe hemorrhage, but ligation will easily control the bleeding.

200 & 201: Questions

200 An eight-year-old, castrated male Irish Setter is presented with sudden onset of abdominal distension and non-productive retching of 2 hours' duration. Physical examination findings are tachycardia, pale gray mucous membranes, prolonged CRT, poor femoral pulse strength, grossly distended abdomen and mildly increased respiratory rate and effort. Your tentative diagnosis is gastric dilatation/volvulus syndrome.
i. What is the most reliable way to make a definitive diagnosis? (Select the best answer.) a. Abdominal ultrasonography. b. Right lateral radiograph of the abdomen. c. Ventrodorsal radiograph of the abdomen. d. Left lateral radiograph of the abdomen.
ii. What is the patient's most life-threatening problem(s) on presentation? (Select the correct answer[s].) a. Hypoventilation due to distended stomach putting pressure on the diaphragm. b. Decreased oxygen delivery due to obstructive, hypovolemic and distributive shock. c. Non-productive retching leading to aspiration pneumonia and sepsis. d. Premature atrial contractions leading to ventricular fibrillation. e. a and b are both correct. f. a and d are both correct. g. All of the above are correct.
iii. What is the most important initial treatment for this dog? (Select the correct answer.) a. Surgery. b. Gastric decompression. c. Mechanical ventilation. d. Large volumes of i/v fluids.
iv. What is the preferred route for administering large volumes of i/v fluids to this 30 kg dog? (Select the correct answer.) a. Through a single large bore catheter in a lateral saphenous vein. b. Through a single long jugular catheter. c. Through two large bore catheters, one in each cephalic vein. d. Through an intraosseous catheter because all the veins are collapsed.
v. What are the most likely arrhythmias to be encountered in this dog postoperatively? (Select the correct answers.) a. Complete atrioventricular dissociation. b. Ventricular escape beats. c. Ventricular premature contractions. d. Electrical mechanical dissociation. e. Premature atrial contractions.

201 A six-year-old, spayed female Springer Spaniel presents with a history of vomiting and diarrhea. HR is 60 bpm; mucous membranes are tacky and pale pink; CRT is 3 seconds. You obtain a stat electrolyte panel which shows: serum potassium – 7.0 mEq/l; sodium – 124 mEq/l; ionized calcium – 3.3 mg/dl (0.82 mmol/l); glucose – 75 mg/dl (4.2 mmol/l).
i. Fill in the following fluid content chart.

Fluid type	Na^+ content	Cl^- content	K^+ content	Ca^{++} content	Buffer type
0.9% NaCl	154				
LRS					Lactate
Plasma-Lyte-A acetate/gluconate			5	0	
1/2 strength LRS with 2.5% dextrose				1.5	
5% dextrose	0				
Hetastarch					
Dextran-70					
Plasma				130	

ii. Based on the chart above, which fluid type would be most appropriate for this patient?
iii. Which fluid type is ideal for free water replacement? Justify your answer.

200 & 201: Answers

200 i. b.
ii. e.
iii. d.
iv. c.
v. c.

201 i.

Fluid type	Na$^+$ content	Cl$^-$ content	K$^+$ content	Ca^{++} content	Buffer type
0.9% NaCl	154	154	0	0	
LRS	130	109	4	3	Lactate
Plasma-Lyte-A acetate/gluconate	140	98	5	0	
1/2 strength LRS with 2.5% dextrose	65	55	2	1.5	Lactate
5% dextrose	0	0	0	0	
Hetastarch	154	154			
Dextran-70	154	154			
Plasma	130	130	<1		

ii. 0.9% sodium chloride would provide fluid for intravascular volume and interstitial replacement without adding potassium.
iii. 5% dextrose is the ideal fluid for free water replacement as this contains no electrolytes, only glucose which is readily metabolized. However, it should not be used as a replacement fluid since it will cause significant intracellular swelling.

202 & 203: Questions

202 This thoracic radiograph (**202**) (Courtesy Dr P Wolvekamp) is of a dog that had tried for an unknown period of time to climb the steep bank of a water filled ditch. When the dog was found by the owner, it was unconscious and not breathing.
i. How would you describe the radiographic abnormalities?
ii. What are the life-threatening events in near-drowning?
iii. What is the first action to be undertaken?
iv. What complications have to be addressed?

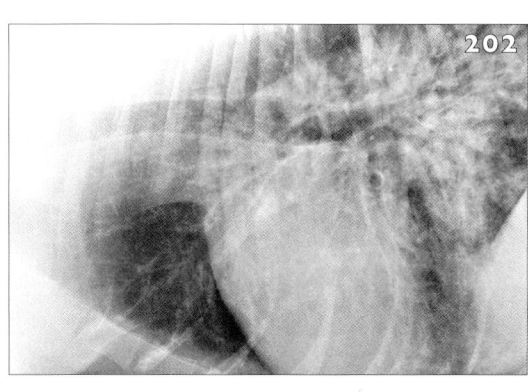

203 A four-year-old, castrated male cat presented after being hit by a car. Initial physical examination findings revealed shock, pallor and pain in the hindquarters or abdomen that was difficult to localize. Initial treatment for shock consisted of i/v crystalloids, supplemental oxygen and analgesic administration. Laboratory evaluation on admission revealed normal values for PCV, TS and creatinine. Blood glucose was 380 mg/dl (21.3 mmol/l). Urine could not be obtained because the urinary bladder was not palpable.
i. What is the most likely explanation for the hyperglycemia in this cat?
   The cat was given fluids and improved initially. However, within 2 hours the cat began vomiting and showed more signs of pain. Repeat physical examination revealed pallor, hypothermia and questionable abdominal distension. At this time it appeared that the cat had normal neurologic function of both hindlimbs. No fractures of long bones or pelvis were palpated. The cat had not produced urine. Red blood was present on the rectal thermometer. Repeat laboratory evaluation revealed low TS, normal PCV, elevated creatinine, normal electrolytes, normal WBC count and hypoglycemia.
ii. What is the likely cause of the deterioration of the cat's condition? (Select the correct answer.) a. Spinal fracture. b. Ruptured urinary bladder. c. Gastrointestinal tract rupture. d. Head trauma. e. b or c.
iii. What would be your next step to assess the cause of the cat's deterioration? (Select the correct answer.) a. Exploratory laparotomy. b. Radiograph the chest and abdomen. c. Abdominocentesis followed by abdominal radiography. d. Obtain an arterial blood gas sample.
iv. Abdominal radiographs were taken and revealed loss of detail, an intact diaphragm and air density between the diaphragm and the liver. What is the radiographic diagnosis and next step? (Select the correct answer.) a. Hydroperitoneum – perform echocardiography. b. Pneumoperitoneum – stabilize and perform abdominal exploratory surgery. c. Uroperitoneum – contrast urethrogram. d. Insufficient information to make a diagnosis.
v. Of all the physical and laboratory parameters given thus far, what is your biggest concern about this patient? (Select the correct answer.) a. Decreased TS. b. Pain. c. Azotemia and lack of urine production. d. Abdominal distension.

202 & 203: Answers

202 i. There is a peribronchial pattern and a diffuse radiodensity with multiple, non-circumscribed, confluent alveolar consolidations in the perihilar region of the caudal lung lobes. The consolidations extend peripherally. Especially in cases of near-drowning, the abnormalities are often in the middle and caudal lung fields. Radiographic abnormalities in the acute stage of near drowning lag behind clinical signs. Ten percent of victims do not aspirate water because of laryngospasm.
ii. Airway obstruction secondary to aspirated material and bronchospasm, pulmonary edema and pulmonary damage due to aspiration of fluids and debris impede ventilation. The dilution of lung surfactant by aspirated water results in alveolar collapse and decreased compliance. The shunting of blood and the ventilation–perfusion mismatch lead to hypoxia. Cardiopulmonary arrest can follow.
iii. Mouth–nose resuscitation should be started as soon as possible after clearing the oral cavity and, if necessary, closed chest cardiac massage should be carried out. Oxygen at 100% is provided after intubation, or as high a concentration as possible if the patient is conscious. In the hospital, mechanical support with positive (end-expiratory) pressure ventilation is often required when pulmonary edema and hypoxia persist.
iv. ARDS can occur secondary to near-drowning and will aggravate pulmonary insufficiency. Specific antibiotic therapy for bacterial pneumonia or abscess formation can be started after diagnosis by means of a tracheal wash. Shock should be treated with i/v fluids. Abnormal consciousness following metabolic stabilization may be the result of cerebral edema and this should be treated by vigorous cerebral resuscitation techniques, including controlled ventilation. Organ failure is anticipated and treated when necessary.

203 i. Most likely stress-induced. The acute neuroendocrine response to trauma involves release of catecholamines, glucocorticoids and glucagon. The net effect of this hormonal response is glycogenolysis, gluconeogenesis, impaired peripheral glucose utilization and inhibition of insulin secretion. Thus blood glucose concentration will rise, especially in the cat.
ii. e.
iii. b.
iv. b.
v. c.

204 & 205: Questions

204 A four-year-old 20 kg male mixed breed dog has been hit by a car. His mucous membranes are pale pink and other vital signs are consistent with hypovolemic compensatory shock. The PCV = 55% and TS = 4.0 g/dl. The dog responds well to your initial resuscitative therapy, but 1 hour later you reassess the patient. You note that the femoral pulses are now weaker, the heart rate is increasing and the abdominal girth has increased. You perform an abdominal centesis and find whole blood (PCV = 30% on the abdominal blood).

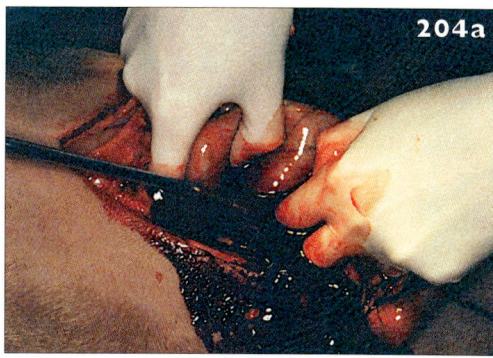
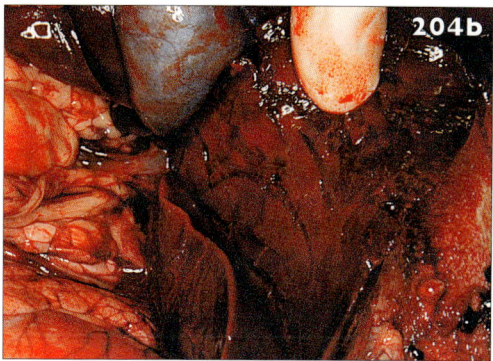

i. Explain the apparent discrepancy between the initial PCV and the initial TS. Discuss appropriate options for fluid resuscitation in this dog.
ii. What steps should you take in the immediate management of this hemoabdomen?
iii. At surgery, you make your abdominal incision and find blood welling up in the peritoneal cavity (**204a**). What will be the most productive way of controlling and localizing the site of hemorrhage?
iv. You discover that there is a badly fractured liver lobe (**204b**). Describe the techniques used in hepatic partial lobectomy.

205 A patient in shock has been on aspirin for 2 months (**205**). This animal requires surgical intervention. What are the pros and cons of using each of the following in this animal?
- Hetastarch
- Dextran-40
- Dextran-70
- Gelatins
- Whole blood

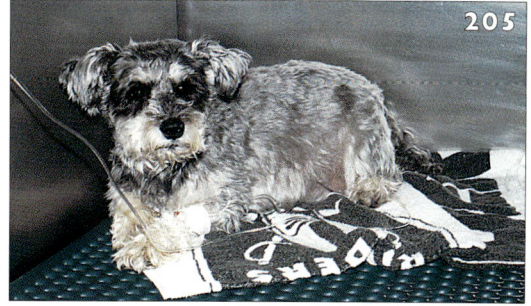

204 & 205: Answers

204 i. Hemorrhage commonly causes a decrease in both the PCV and TS due to loss of both RBCs and proteins. However, in shock the PCV may be elevated due to the shock response of splenic contraction seen in the dog. Both PCV and TS will drop due to dilution if crystalloid fluids with or without synthetic colloids to restore circulating volume. With crystalloids alone, the serum oncotic pressure will fall as the TS falls. A combination of crystalloids and colloids is ideal. Should bleeding become significant, whole blood is the colloid of choice. Hypertonic saline (7.5%) could be used with the crystalloids and colloids during the initial fluid resuscitation. When intracavity bleeding is suspected, hypotensive resuscitation is employed. This means that the patient is only resuscitated to normal or slightly below normal blood pressures to avoid dislodging the protective clot as blood pressures elevate.

ii. Binding of the rear limbs and abdomen can help to tamponade a bleeding abdomen and redistribute systemic circulation to more anterior vital organs. As blood is being administered, the animal is prepared for surgical exploration.

iii. Attempting to suction all blood from the peritoneal cavity until the site of hemorrhage can be visualized is generally unsuccessful and can contribute to the exsanguination and death of the patient. The bleeding will continue until stopped by ligation or pressure. A small abdominal incision is made and the hand slides down the abdominal wall back to the aorta, anterior to the celiac artery The cranial abdominal aorta is digitally compressed at this site and the abdomen is packed with surgical towels. Once packed, the cranial abdominal aorta is visualized and a temporary vascular nare is place around it. Then, quadrant by quadrant, the packs are removed and the area explored for bleeding. When all sources of bleeding are temporarily controlled, you can begin definitive repair with ligation or excision. The aorta may be occluded for no longer than 15 minutes without serious risk of spinal cord necrosis. Partial splenectomy or hepatic lobectomy may be necessary.

iv. Gentle finger pressure is used to bluntly fracture the affected lobe proximal to the non-viable or damaged portion of the lobe. Your fracture line should expose all vessels and ducts and these should subsequently be securely ligated. The choice of suture for ligatures is largely dictated by the surgeon's preference, although vascular clips or staples provide a quick method. It is not necessary to oversew the raw edge of the liver lobe.

205

• *Hetastarch* – Effectively increases circulating volume. However, it will not improve platelet function. Hetastarch infusion above the recommended dose can increase bleeding times in the surgical patient.

• *Dextran-40 and -70* – Will increase circulating volume but they coat the platelets and depress platelet bridging. This factor is important in a surgical patient on aspirin.

• *Gelatins* – Effectively increase circulating volume. While providing no improvement in the hemostatic ability of the patient, the gelatins do not interfere with coagulation.

• *Whole blood* – Stored whole blood has no viable platelets, but would be an effective volume expander if this patient lost blood. Fresh whole blood would be the ideal volume expander for a surgical patient with decreased platelet function, as it would supply a moderate amount of functional platelets while providing circulatory volume and RBCs during blood loss.

206 & 207: Questions

206 This four-year old female miniature Schnauzer with a history of immune-mediated hemolytic anemia becomes acutely tachypneic (**206**).
i. Give two probable reasons for the dyspnea seen in this patient.
ii. Describe your diagnostic plan to determine the etiology of the tachypnea.
iii. Describe your treatment of this patient's respiratory distress.

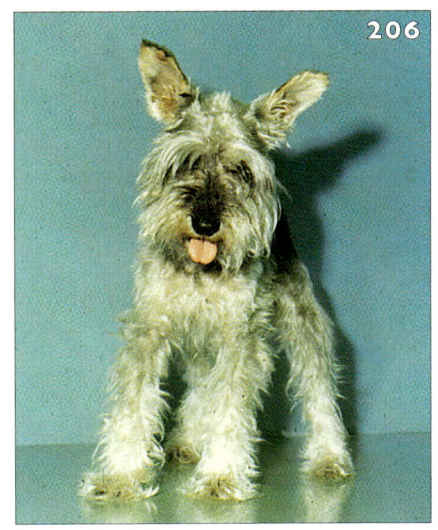

207 A male Bernese Mountain Dog, aged nine, was presented to the emergency service with a mild lameness of 2 months' duration and an acute non-weightbearing lameness after running. Orthopedic examination revealed a painful left proximal radius and ulna with firm soft tissue swelling.
i. What is the radiological interpretation (**206**)?
ii. What are the differential diagnoses?
iii. What further diagnostic tests should be carried out and what would be your initial treatment, regardless of the underlying cause?
iv. What is the prognosis?

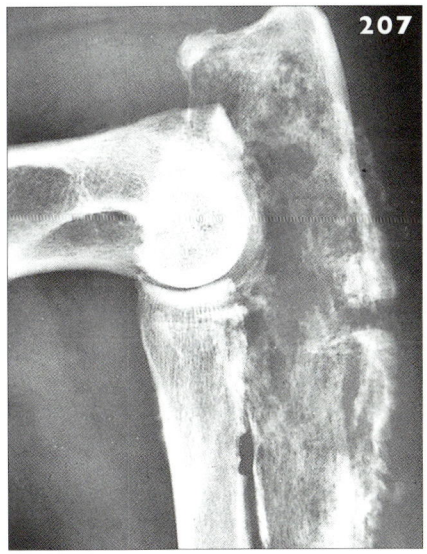

206 & 207: Answers

206 i. Two differentials for acute onset of dyspnea in a dog with IMHA are pulmonary thromboembolism (PTE) and severe anemia.
ii. The first step in determining the cause of this patient's tachypnea is to evaluate the PCV. If the PCV is stable and has not acutely decreased, then anemia is unlikely to be the cause of tachypnea. Diagnosing the presence of PTE is more difficult. Evaluation of an arterial blood gas will reveal the presence of hypoxemia with normal ventilation. Repeating the arterial blood gas evaluation with the patient receiving supplemental oxygen will determine if the hypoxemia is oxygen responsive. Thoracic radiographs are not helpful in confirming the presence of PTE. Confirming the presence of PTE will require the use of nuclear scintigraphy or angiography.
iii. The dog should immediately be given oxygen supplementation. If the tachypnea is found to be due to severe anemia, administration of a whole blood transfusion or packed red cells may be necessary. If PTE is suspected, the patient should be started on heparin therapy to prevent the formation of further thrombi. Aspirin therapy should also be considered. Administration of vitamin K antagonists such as coumadin may be necessary to prolong the PT and prevent further thrombi formation. Thrombolytic agents such as streptokinase or urokinase may also be used.

207 i. There are severe osteolytic changes in the proximal ulna and a fracture line can be observed within the osteolytic zone. There is a rough periosteal surface on the ulna. The radial and humeral bone on this view seem not involved.
ii. a. Osteogenic tumor with pathological fracture, probably osteosarcoma, rule out chondro- and fibrosarcoma and secondary bone tumors. b. Fungal osteomyelitis (unlikely and only regionally important).
iii. Pain relief with pain medication and supportive bandage. Skeletal tumor pain is considered severe, opioid analgesia is indicated. Oxymorphone or transdermal fentanyl patches are good choices of analgesics. A clinical staging to rule out the presence of metastatic disease should be performed as soon as possible. It includes basic lab work, a thorough physical and orthopedic exam with survey films of the skeleton and thoracic x-rays to rule out macroscopic pulmonary metastasis. The working diagnosis of osteosarcoma should be confirmed either with a core biopsy with a 'Jamshidi' needle or, in this case, together with an amputation of the foreleg to evaluate the mass *in toto*. Limb-sparing surgery is possible: it would include a very difficult fusion of the elbow joint. Cisplatin chemotherapy is indicated in the treatment of osteosarcoma with either amputation or limb-sparing surgery.
iv. If this is a tumor, poor. Dogs treated with amputation alone have a median survival time of 25 weeks and those treated with amputation and chemotherapy have been shown to have a median survival time of 43 weeks.

208–210: Questions

208 A male Rottweiler, four months old, was presented to the emergency service. The physical examination was normal but the orthopedic examination revealed a non-weightbearing lameness of the right hindleg. Palpation of the right hindleg revealed pain in the knee joint, but the knee itself had no increase in drawer motion and there was no crepitation. No joint effusion could be seen or palpated.
i. What is the radiological interpretation (**208**)?
ii. How can you confirm the diagnosis?
iii. Surgical repair is indicated. Why?
iv. What is the postoperative management? Describe the long-term problems with this diagnosis.

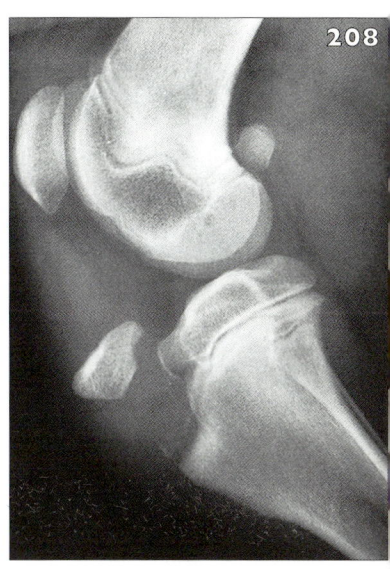

209 This spleen (**209**) was taken from an eleven-year-old Golden Retriever with a palpable abdominal mass and an abdominal fluid wave. He had a heart rate of 180 bpm, CRT of 3 sec, pale mucous membranes, and femoral pulses that were hardly palpable. Initial data base revealed a PCV of 30%; TS = 3.0 g/dl.
i. What is the most ideal colloid solution used during resuscitation and why?
ii. During fluid resuscitation of this patient, what parameters should be closely monitored and why?
iii. What is the definitive treatment for volume control in this patient?

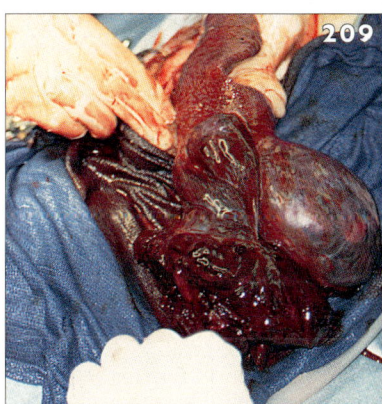

210 Twenty minutes after being hit by a car, a two-year-old intact male Labrador Retriever is presented. Physical examination reveals a respiratory rate of 60 breaths/minute, heart rate of 180bpm, pale mucous membranes, weak pulses and a tense painful abdomen. Abdominocentesis (**210**) reveals a hemorrhagic fluid.
i. How would you confirm your suspicions of hemoabdomen?
ii In your initial workup, PCV is 25% but the anemia appears non-regenerative. Why is that?
iii. Following administration of 45 ml/kg of crystalloids, PCV = 15% and TS = 3.2 g/dl. Describe your choice of fluid and the method of blood collection and transfusion.

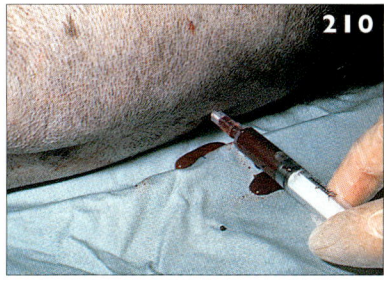

208–210: Answers

208 i. Avulsion of the tibial crest.
ii. Try to elicit painful palpation on extension of the stifle; soft tissue swelling and crepitus might be present. If the displaced tibial crest is located above the proximal tibial epiphyseal plate an avulsion can usually be diagnosed without additional x-rays. If the findings are not clear, compare x-rays of the contralateral side.
iii. The tibial crest is the insertion of the straight patellar tendon and therefore the insertion of the quadriceps apparatus. A partial loss of function is present with avulsion of the insertion. The extension of the leg is particularly limited without proper fixation of the tibial crest.
iv. Because of the 'minimal fixation' devices used to keep the avulsed crest at its physiological position, it is necessary to restrict movement of the leg with a Robert Jones bandage for at least 10 days. Interference with normal epiphyseal growth is possible especially if the fixation devices are not removed shortly after healing is evident. The animal should be fully weightbearing and should be free of pain on palpation before implants can be removed.

209 i. Whole blood is the ideal resuscitation fluid, along with an isotonic crystalloid fluid. There is evidence of blood loss, as indicated by the PCV/TS, and of poor perfusion, as indicated by prolonged CRT, pale mucous membranes and poor pulse strength.
ii. Blood pressure, PCV/TS, gum color, heart rate, and abdominal size are closely monitored. Evidence of hypotension and poor perfusion that persists in spite of resuscitation, or recurs after resuscitation, implies ongoing abdominal hemorrhage.
iii. This patient requires surgical intervention for ultimate hemostasis and volume control.

210 i. The first step in determining the origin of the abdominal fluid should be to determine the fluid's PCV. If the PCV is consistent with blood, there are two major differentials for its source: free blood within the abdominal cavity or blood from the puncture of a peripheral vessel or vascular organ such as the liver or spleen. If the blood retrieved by abdominocentesis truly reflects the presence of a hemoabdomen, the retrieved blood will not clot. If, however, the blood retrieved is the result of puncture of the spleen, liver or a peripheral vessel, this blood should clot. The presence of free blood within the abdominal cavity results in defibrination of the blood, the result being no clot.
ii. Typically, anemia associated with blood loss is regenerative. However, evidence of a regenerative response is not present in the peripheral blood for 3–4 days after blood loss.
iii. With an acute drop in PCV and TS, administration of whole blood transfusion should be considered. If the patient has been previously transfused or it appears that multiple transfusions may be necessary (and when time allows) the patient is cross-matched with potential donors in order to decrease the incidence of transfusion reactions. Once a suitable donor is found, fresh blood can be drawn or stored whole blood can be administered. Canine whole blood drawn in CPD-A1 can be stored for 25–32 days at –1 to –6°C. Heparin should not be routinely used as an anticoagulant in tranfusion administration as it readily activates platelets and has no preservative characteristics. If heparin is used in blood intended for transfusion (625 units heparin/50 ml whole blood), the blood must be administered within 48 hours.

The volume and rate of blood administered varies with the patient's clinical signs and laboratory data. In this case, enough whole blood should be administered to alleviate the patient's signs of anemia. In general, 2 ml/kg of whole blood will increase the patient's PCV by 1%. The transfusion rate for whole blood should be 5 ml/kg during a 4-hour period or, if the patient is hypovolemic, 5 ml/kg/hr. The first 10 ml should be given slowly over a 15 minute period to check for adverse reactions. Blood should be administered through an appropriate filter and administration set designed to retain clots and debris. Should the patient require blood immediately, an autotransfusion of the abdominal blood can be given.

211 & 212: Questions

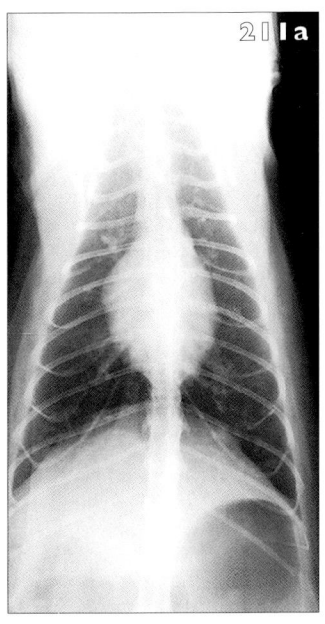
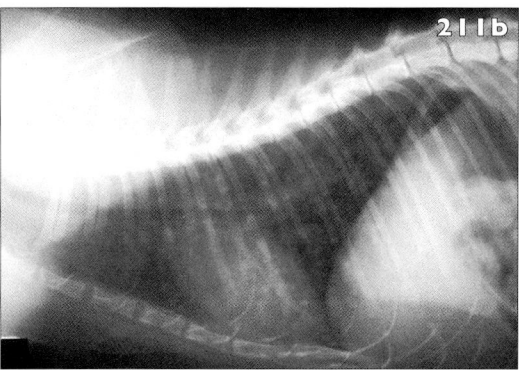

211 A five-year-old neutered male Siamese cat is presented after several hours of progressive dyspnea. There are no auscultable murmurs or arrhythmias. The cat is tachypneic but stable enough for thoracic radiographs.
i. Describe the radiographic findings. What disease process do these radiographs (211a, 211b) suggest?
ii. What additional diagnostic tests would help to further characterize this condition?
iii. Describe the cellular findings expected from the airway with this diagnosis.
iv. What is your therapeutic plan?

212 A two-year-old female ferret presents with multiple vomiting episodes. A firm mass is palpated in the abdomen. Radiographs reveal a radio-opaque mass in the intestines with an obstructive gas pattern (212).

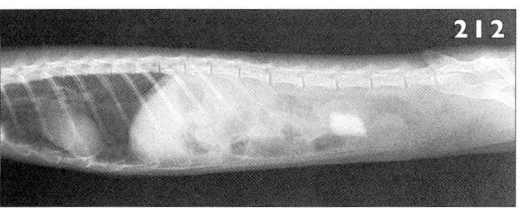

i. Describe a systematic approach for exploration in the abdomen.
ii. If there is questionable bowel viability in intestines with an apparently intact wall, what procedure can be performed to rule out significant transmural leakage of the bowel contents?
iii. How can strictures of the intestinal lumen be prevented when removing single foreign objects without requiring anastamosis?

211 & 212: Answers

211 i. The radiographs (**211a, 211b**) demonstrate peribronchial densities, hyperlucency of the lung fields and flattening of the diaphragm, suggesting hyperinflation. The gas-filled stomach is evidence of aerophagia. The presence of infiltrates around the small airways in all lung fields is characteristic of allergic bronchial disease (i.e. feline asthma). Magnification of the peripheral airways would reveal 'donuts' and 'tramlines' formed by lucent central airways surrounded by opaque peribronchial infiltrates.

ii. A complete blood count should be performed to evaluate signs of infectious disease or peripheral eosinophilia. A transtracheal aspirate sample should be examined carefully for cell morphology, as well as for parasite ova and larvae or fungal organisms, and should also be submitted for bacterial culture and antibiotic sensitivity testing. There should be a fecal examination for parasites, which should include fecal flotation (for *Capillaria* and *Toxoplasma*), Baermann technique (for *Aelurostrongylus*), and sedimentation (for *Paragonimus*). An occult heartworm test is also indicated. Extended discussion with the owners may determine a possible antigen or irritant exposure (i.e. smoking, new litter or other aerosols in the home).

iii. The tracheobronchial wash sample in a cat with feline asthma typically contains a mixed population of inflammatory cells (nondegenerate neutrophils, eosinophils, macrophages). Although this could represent a number of infectious or inflammatory disorders, it is suggestive of allergic bronchitis or feline asthma.

iv. The initial plan includes oxygen supplementation, methylxanthines (aminophylline 5 mg/kg slowlyi/v, i/m or p/o), terbutaline (0.625 mg p/o or 0.1 mg s/c or nebulized), steroids (prednisolone sodium succinate 5–100 mg/cat i/v once, dexamethasone 0.05–0.1 mg/kg i/m, s/c), and, in cases of severe distress, sympathomimetics (epinephrine 0.1 mg s/c)

Chronic management should include steroid therapy (prednisolone 0.5–1.0 mg/kg/day, tapered to lowest effective dose, or methylprednisolone acetate 2–4 mg/kg i/m every 10–30 days), bronchodilators (aminophylline 5 mg/kg p/o bid, theophylline 4 mg/kg p/o bid, terbutaline 0.625 mg p/o bid), and removal of suspected antigens (i.e. dusty kitty litter, talc, cigarette smoke).

212 i. The most important aspect is a detailed and consistent approach in inspecting all organs. One method is to start with the gastrointestinal tract, looking at the esophageal hiatus, follow the stomach both ventrally and dorsally, inspect the pylorus, follow the duodenum as it passes across to the left side of the abdomen, run the small bowel from jejunum to ileum, at the same time inspecting the mesenteric vessels and lymph nodes. The ileocecal junction and colon is followed into the pelvic inlet. The diaphragm and peritoneal wall is then inspected and palpated for tension/masses. All lobes of the liver are inspected as well as the gall bladder and ducts. The pancreas is inspected with minimal manipulation. The spleen is gently pulled out of the celomic cavity and inspected, with the hilar vessels palpated for pulsations. The right kidney and ureter are exposed by lifting the descending portion of the duodenum, positioning the remaining loops of intestine to the left of the mesoduodenum. The left kidney and ureter are exposed by lifting the descending colon and mesentery, displacing the loops of bowel to the right. The ureters are followed to their insertion in the neck of the bladder. The bladder is inspected. Any genital organs present are then inspected.

ii. A sterile swab of the serosa of the questionable bowel is prepared for intraoperative cytological evaluation. Any evidence of bacteria or fiber contents suggests migration or leakage of chyme and the area should be resected.

iii. The longitudinal incision of the enterotomy is closed transversely with a simple interrupted pattern.

213 & 214: Questions

213 An eight-year-old male Labrador was presented to the emergency service with a history of a fracture repair 2 months prior to presentation of the left tibia. He was acutely lame before presentation. **213a** shows a post-operative view of the fracture repair and **213b** is a radiograph taken at the emergency hospital 2 months later.
i. What is your radiographic interpretation?
ii. Explain the biomechanics of this implant failure and its consequences.
iii. What treatment would you prescribe?

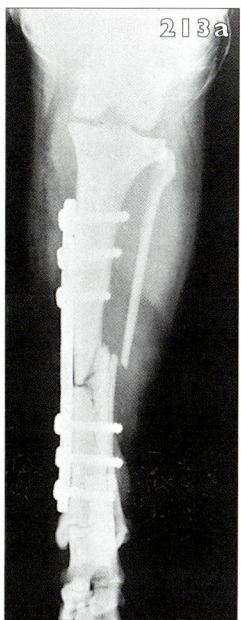
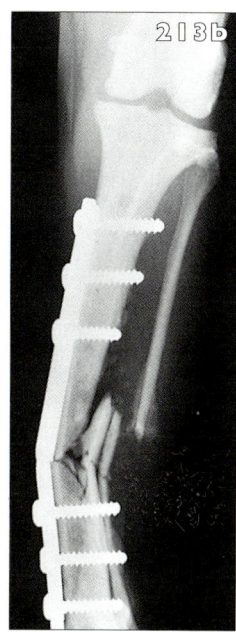

214 This six-year-old 13 kg male intact cryptorchid Schnauzer is presented for weakness, lethargy, intermittent epistaxis and melena of 1 week's duration. Physical findings include gynecomastia, a pendulous prepuce, symmetrical truncal alopecia, a papable mid-abdominal mass, pale mucous membranes and a fever of 103.5°F (39.7°C). The dog's hematocrit is 14%, with a total protein of 7.0 g/dl. A blood smear reveals normocytic, normochromic anemia with a platelet count of 6000/mm³. The white blood cell count is 2500/mm³.

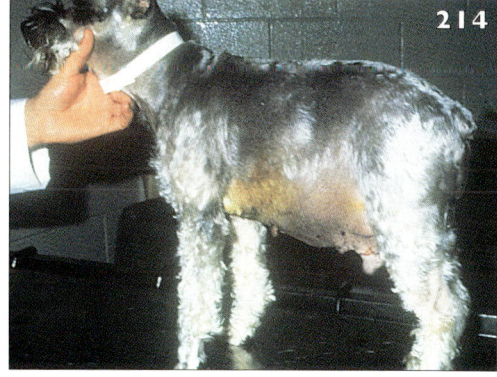

i. What is your presumptive diagnosis?
ii. If you gave this dog a blood transfusion, how much blood would you give him?
iii. What are your treatment recommendations?

213 & 214: Answers

213 i. Broken boneplate, fracture nonunion with bending of the tibial repair in the direction of the long axis, possible bony sequester formation on the medial side of the fracture.
ii. The initial fracture consists of a comminuted tibial fracture with a laterally (transcortical) located free fragment. The initial fracture fixation did not include the reconstruction and stable fixation of the lateral aspect of the fracture leading to missing lateral support of this fracture. The axial load of the tibia is therefore almost totally absorbed by the plate. The neutral axis becomes centered within the plate. The plate is under more bending stress which can increase to the point of breakage of the plate.
iii. Plate removal, biopsy and culture to rule out a coexisting osteomyelitis of the fracture site, assessment of viability of the questionable bone fragments, stable internal fixation with another bone plate and lag screw fixation of the lateral free fragment if considered a viable fragment during surgery to support the lateral side (transcortex). External fixation with a rigid external fixator would be an alternative, plate removal and evaluation of the fracture would still be necessary.

214 i. Cryptorchid dogs are prone to testicular tumors. This dog has an estrogen-secreting tumor (Sertoli cell tumor or seminoma) which is causing the clinical signs of male feminization and bone marrow suppression.
ii. If we wanted to raise this dog's hematocrit to 30% and the hematocrit of the donor blood was 45%, we could use the following formula to determine the amount of blood to transfuse.

$$\text{\#ml blood needed} = \frac{(\text{HCT desired}) - (\text{HCT actual})}{(\text{HCT donor})} \times \text{BW kg} \times \frac{90 \text{ ml}}{\text{kg}}$$

$$= \frac{(30 - 14)}{45} \times 13 \text{ kg} \times \frac{90 \text{ ml}}{\text{kg}} = 416 \text{ ml}$$

Fresh whole blood should be used to supply platelets as well as red blood cells. Platelet-rich plasma may be needed to supply additional platelets if hemorrhage is a problem.
iii. The prognosis for this dog is guarded to poor because of the bone marrow suppression affecting all three cell lines. The only hope for a reversal of bone marrow suppression is the removal of the source of estrogen secretion. The dog should be stabilized with a transfusion as described above and treated with intravenous bactericidal antibiotics before surgical removal of the tumor. Removal of gastrointestinal parasites may decrease platelet consumption and blood loss through melena. Reversal of aplastic anemia may take several months, during which time the dog must be supported with transfusions and control of infections as needed. Erythropoeitin (l00 U/kg s/c three times a week) is generally not useful in stimulating red blood cell production because endogenous erythropoeitin production is already adequate in these patients. Recombinant canine granulocyte colony stimulating factor (rcG-CSF) has been cloned, but is not yet commercially available. A dosage of 5 µg/kg/day s/c effectively raises white blood cell counts and has not been associated with toxicity. Human recombinant granulocyte colony stimulating factor can induce neutropenia as a result of antibody formation against foreign G-CSF and it should be used only on a short-term basis or not at all.

215 & 216: Questions

215 A nine-month-old spayed female mixed-breed dog was struck by an automobile about 30 minutes prior to presentation. Voluntary motor function was present in the pelvic limbs but the dog could not stand. A preoperative lateral spinal radiograph (**215a**) shows the spinal injury. The surgical repair is illustrated in the postoperative radiograph (**215b**).
i. Describe the spinal injury shown in the preoperative radiograph.
ii. What spinal cord segments are normally located in the canine spinal canal at the fractured vertebra?
iii. What biomaterials have been used to stabilize the fracture?
iv. Spinal fractures are divided into dorsal and ventral spinal column compartment injuries to facilitate decisions on which fractures are unstable enough to warrant surgical stabilization. Which compartment is stabilized by the fixation in this dog?
v. Why would vertebral body-plating be undesirable for this fracture?
vi. In general, injury to which spinal column compartment results in more instability?
vii. Anatomically, what constitutes the dorsal and ventral spinal column compartments?

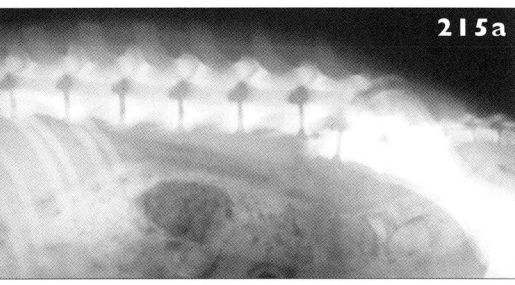
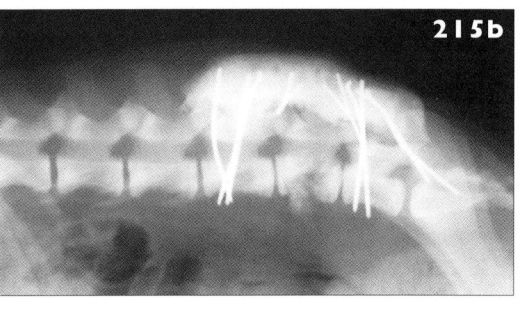

216 A four-year-old, castrated male Schnauzer is presented after it had been rescued from a house fire. On presentation the dog has a RR of 45 bpm, with an increased inspiratory effort and moderate distress (**216**).
i. The dog's mucous membranes are bright red. What is the significance of this observation?
ii. What is your initial therapeutic plan?
iii. What complications should you anticipate, and how would you monitor for them?

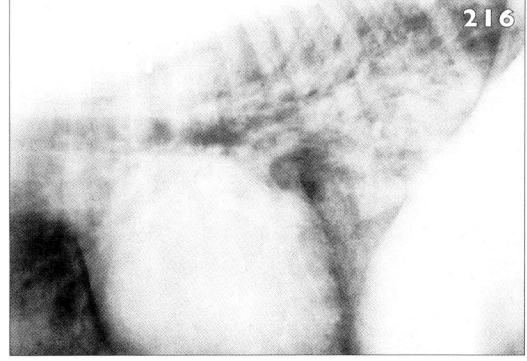

215 & 216: Answers

215 i. A comminuted oblique fracture of the body of L6 with approximately 150% displacement of the spinal canal is seen on the radiograph.
ii. The coccygeal (caudal) spinal cord segments are normally found at the location of the fractured vertebra.
iii. Polymethylmethacrylate and stainless steel pins have been used in this stabilization procedure.
iv. The ventral compartment has been stabilized in this dog.
v. Vertebral body plating requires rhizotomy. In this case rhizotomy of L5 and L6 nerve roots would result in some lower motor neuron limb dysfunction.
vi. Injury to the ventral compartment causes more spinal column instability than does injury to the dorsal compartment.
vii. The dorsal spinal column compartment consists of:
• Laminae and pedicles.
• Dorsal spinous processes.
• Articular facets and joint capsules.
• Supraspinous/interspinous ligaments.
The ventral spinal column compartment consists of:
• Vertebral bodies.
• Intervertebral discs.
• Dorsal and ventral longitudinal ligaments.
• Transverse processes.

216 i. The bright red mucous membranes suggest carbon monoxide toxicity. Carbon monoxide displaces oxygen on hemoglobin molecules, forming carboxyhemoglobin complexes and leading to tissue hypoxia.
ii. Supplementation with 100% oxygen reduces the half-life of the carboxyhemoglobin complexes from 4 hours ($t_{1/2}$ on room air) to 30 minutes. Oxygen should be humidified to promote mucociliary clearance and prevent drying injuries to the airways. Steroids are contraindicated unless severe edema and upper airway swelling exist. Smoke inhalation patients may also have significant cutaneous burns as well, and they should be treated aggressively with i/v fluids, wound care and nutritional support.
iii. Heat injuries to upper airways can lead to swelling, edema, laryngeal spasm and potentially to upper airway obstruction. Irritation from smoke and hot particles can promote the development of ARDS and decrease mucociliary function, thus predisposing the victim to developing bronchopneumonia.

217 & 218: Questions

217 This five-year-old domestic shorthair cat (**217**) was presented to the emergency hospital with a penetrating knife injury.
i. What should your telephone instructions be to owners whose pets are impaled?
ii. How would you evaluate the extent or path of this injury? (Select the best answer.)
a. Complete physical exam.
b. Radiographs of the affected area.
c. Rectal exam.
d. Surgical exploration.
e. All of the above.
iii. Which of the following should **not** be done by the veterinarian when treating this wound?
a. Remove the knife.
b. Institute antibiotic therapy.
c. Lavage with 5% providone-iodine solution.
d. Surgically debride necrotic and contaminated tissue.

218 A ten-year-old dog presents for twice vomiting yellow foam and reluctance to stand. Physical examination found the dog to have normal vital signs, thoracic auscultation and abdominal palpation. The dog's hips were sore on rotation and abduction. Neurological examination showed the dog to have a left-sided head tilt and horizontal nystagmus, and a fast phase to the left that remained the same in all body positions. The dog had a ventral strabismus in the right eye when the nose was elevated straight upward. Other cranial nerves were normal. The dog had an ataxic gait but the front and rear limb

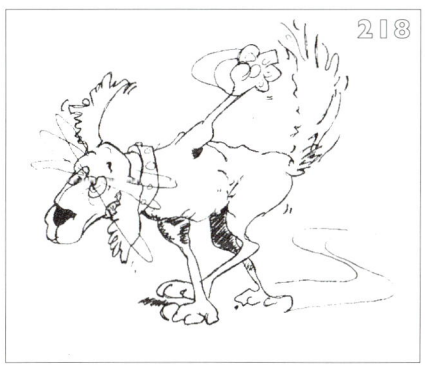

flexor reflexes were normal. It had the same strength when hemistanding and hemiwalking on the right and the left. Conscious proprioception was normal in all four limbs.
i. Which system within the nervous system is most likely affected?
ii. Is a head tilt usually toward or away from the site of the lesion?
iii. The pathology can occur in two general locations in relation to the central nervous system: name them.
iv. Describe some signs seen on neurologic examination that help to differentiate the two general locations.
v. Why is it important to try to differentiate these two locations?
vi. In which of the two locations is this dog's lesion most likely to be and why?
vii. What symptomatic therapy may be of some benefit?
viii. What specific therapy will be of benefit?
ix. What prognosis do you give to this owner?

217 & 218: Answers

217 i. Owners should be advised to greatly restrain or immobilize the pet during transport. Foreign objects such as knives should be removed only by the veterinarian. Long arrow shafts protruding from the wound can be shortened with bolt cutters as long as the point of the arrow is stabilized.
ii. e. A complete physical exam, radiographs of the affected area and examination of the entire path at the time of surgery have obvious value. In this area, a rectal exam is a rapid test and would be extremely important in determining whether the knife had penetrated the rectum or colon. Wounds penetrating the abdomen should be explored as soon as the cat has been stabilized.
iii. c. 3–5% providone-iodine solution is toxic to fibroblasts. Also, iodine can be absorbed into the systemic circulation.

218 i. Vestibular system.
ii. Toward the side of the lesion.
iii. Central or peripheral nervous systems. Peripheral cranial nerve VIII or central brainstem near the VIIIth nucleus or in the flocculonodular lobe of the cerebellum.
iv *Either:* head tilt; horizontal nystagmus; rotatory nystagmus; ataxia; nystagmus does not change with body positioning; and vomiting.
Central: other cranial nerve signs along with hemiparesis or conscious proprioception deficits; cerebellar signs; vertical nystagmus; positional nystagmus; paradoxical head tilt.
Peripheral: can have cranial nerve VII and Horner's syndrome with middle ear infection or trauma; long tract signs will, however, be normal.
v. Peripheral lesions in animals can be due to middle ear infections or trauma; in older dogs, idiopathic peripheral vestibular disease occurs; both have good prognoses. Central disease has a serious list of potential etiologies and carries a grave prognosis, warranting aggressive diagnostic testing.
vi. Peripheral is most likely, due to the lack of long tract or cerebellar signs.
vii. Antihistamines or other motion-sickness medications may help relieve the nausea; if the dog is rolling, a tranquilizer such as diazepam can give some relief.
viii. Treat any signs of middle ear infection. There is no specific therapy for neurological signs.
ix. Good, unless the neurological signs change.

219 & 220: Questions

219 A five-year-old female spayed cat is presented unconsious after being hit by a car 30 minutes earlier. The cat has been unconscious since the accident.
i. List the five levels of consciousness.
ii. What is the system within the brain responsible for consciousness and where is it located?
iii. Define stupor. Define coma. Which of the two has a better overall prognosis?
iv. A neurological examination is carried out to try to localize the lesion – to what two main areas of the brain?

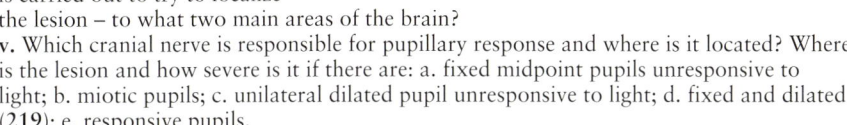

v. Which cranial nerve is responsible for pupillary response and where is it located? Where is the lesion and how severe is it if there are: a. fixed midpoint pupils unresponsive to light; b. miotic pupils; c. unilateral dilated pupil unresponsive to light; d. fixed and dilated (**219**); e. responsive pupils.
vi. Which parts of the brain are functioning normally to provide a normal nystagmus that is induced by horizontal or vertical movement of the head? What is the caloric test?
vii. What is decerebrate rigidity and why does it occur?

220 A 13-year-old, male Cocker Spaniel presents with severe dyspnea (80 bpm) and periodic coughing of blood-tinged frothy fluid. HR is 160 bpm, pulses are very weak, a gallop is auscultated and mucous membranes are very pale with cyanosis. The dog's history includes a previous diagnosis of congestive heart failure secondary to mitral valvular endocardiosis associated with a grade V/VI

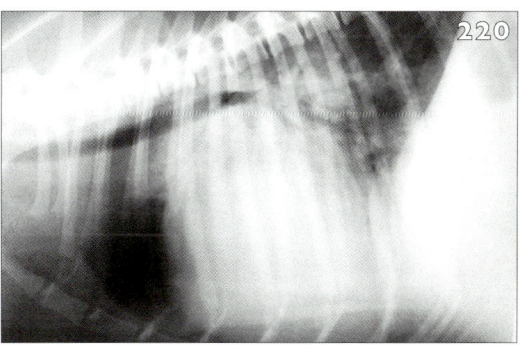

murmur. His current medications include enalapril, furosemide and digoxin.
i. After 0.5 inch (2 cm) nitroglycerin, two doses of furosemide (75 mg i/v), enalapril and oxygen, you obtain chest radiographs but have to return the dog to oxygen immediately due to cyanosis. What is your interpretation of the radiograph (**220**), and your assessment of the patient?
ii. What additional drug therapy would you include in this patient at this time?
iii. How would you monitor this patient?
iv. What is the significance of the gallop auscultated?

219 & 220: Answers

219 i. Alert, depressed, delirium, stupor, coma.
ii. The ascending reticular activating system receives sensory input from the periphery and runs from the reticular formation to the thalamus and then to the cerebral cortex.
iii. Stupor is the level of consciousness when the animal is unconsious but arousable with a noxious stimulus. Coma is the level of consciousness when the animal is unconscious and not arousable with any stimulus. Stupor has a better overall prognosis than coma.
iv. Diffuse cerebral cortex or midbrain/brain stem.
v. The third cranial nerve, located in the midbrain, is responsible for pupillary constriction. The sympathetic nerve is responsible for pupillary dilation.
a. If the pupils are fixed in midpoint position and unresponsive to light, a midbrain lesion is suspected and the prognosis should be considered guarded.
b. Miotic pupils can be associated with cerebral, diencephalic or pontine lesions and can have a better prognosis.
c. A unilateral dilated pupil unresponsive to light is associated with oculomotor nerve lesions and can be due to cerebral swelling and occipital lobe herniation under the tentorium cerebelli.
d. Pupils fixed and dilated are suggestive of midbrain disease.
e. Responsive pupils carry a better prognosis and imply cerebral origin of altered consciousness.
vi. The presence of normal vestibular nystagmus seen on movement of the head horizontally and vertically indicates the brain is intact from the rostral medulla to the midbrain. The ear canal can be irrigated with hot water (caloric test) and if horizontal nystagmus is induced, the brain stem is intact as well.
vii. Extension of the head, neck and limbs in the unconscious patient is generally decerebrate rigidity, due to compression of the red nucleus within the midbrain, thereby removing the flexor input to the body.

220 i. Marked cardiomegaly with an alveolar and interstitial pattern compatible with pulmonary edema. Decompensating congestive heart failure is likely.
ii. Addition of a thiazide diuretic alone may improve response. However, with a refractory heart failure secondary to mitral regurgitation, hydralazine (0.5 mg/kg p/o) or, alternatively, an i/v nitroprusside infusion (a potent arteriolar dilator and venodilator) is likely to be effective.
iii. At a respiration rate <50 bpm, a maintenance dose of furosomide can be instituted. With hydralazine or nitroprusside, BP monitoring is essential. A baseline MAP or a systolic BP are obtained, then repeated in 1 hour.
iv. In congestive heart failure the ventricle becomes less compliant and more stiff. Typically, when the ventricle is dilated a low-intensity S_3 gallop sound is best heard with the bell of the stethoscope placed over the left ventricular apex.

221 & 222: Questions

221 Amber is a five-year-old (40 kg) intact female Golden Retriever that presented for abdominal pain, vomiting, and sanguinous discharge from her vulva. She has been anorexic and very depressed for 1 day. Physical examination found: T = 102.4°F (39.1°C); HR = 160 bpm; RR = 25 bpm; mucous membrane = hyperemic

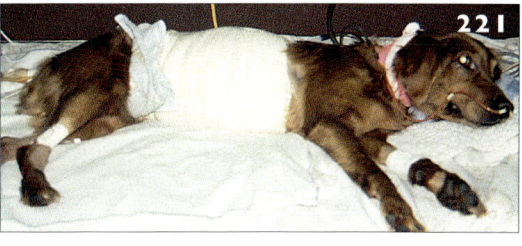

and dry; CRT = 1 sec; femoral pulses were weak; mentally depressed and weak; bloody vaginal discharge; generalized pain on abdominal palpation; thoracic auscultation was normal. The dog was estimated to be 8% dehydrated.
i. What is the perfusion status of this dog? What physical parameters do you use to evaluate this? What physical parameters do you use to assess for hydration status? Perfusion deficits are in which fluid compartment? Dehydration is due to a deficit in which fluid compartment?
ii. What aspect of the physical examination of this dog gives you a good indication that this will not be an 'uncomplicated' pyometra? What is a likely etiology for these changes on physical examination?
The initial laboratory work revealed: WBC = 2500/mm^3 (80% mature neutrophils); PCV = 54%; TS = 8.2 g/dl; BUN labstick = 30–40 mg/dl; glucose labstick = 120 mg/dl (6.72 mmol/l); Na$^+$ = 148 mEq/l; K$^+$ = 3.4 mEq/l; ACT = 100 sec; platelet count = 150,000/mm^3; ATIII = 67%; urinalysis: specific gravity = 1.020; 2+ protein, 3+ blood. Radiographs of the abdomen reveal enlarged tubular structures in the caudal abdomen and a mild loss of detail in the caudal and mid-abdomen.
iii. Give your assessment of the laboratory work.
iv. Give your initial resuscitation plan for this dog.
v. When would you take this dog to surgery and why?
At surgery, the dog had an enlarged uterus with purulent exudate leaking into the abdomen from the fallopian tube.
vi. What are some specific surgical considerations once these abnormalities are noted?
vii. List 20 parameters (Rule of 20) that must be carefully assessed and monitored in this animal to ensure an optimal outcome.

222 The scene is the waiting room of an emergency clinic on a busy Sunday afternoon. The veterinary nurse is called to triage five walk-in cases:
a. A five-year-old dog that has had two seizures since last night, the last one was 4 hours ago.
b. A 12-year-old, spayed female cat that 'is not acting right' for the last 8 hours. The cat has rapid shallow breathing and is reluctant to lie down.
c. A three-year-old German Shepherd Dog with a 1 inch (2.5 cm) laceration to the dorsal aspect of its right front metacarpal region. The owners have placed a compression bandage.
d. An 18-year-old, castrated male Shetland Sheepdog presented dead on arrival.
e. A one-year-old Labrador 'extremely hyper' for the last 2 hours. The dog was outside unobserved for 3 hours prior to onset of signs. The dog is mildly excited with intermittent episodes of mental dullness.
  Utilizing the principles of triage, how should the nurse prioritize these patients?

221 & 222: Answers

221 i. This dog is in the compensatory stage of shock. Perfusion parameters are assessed by heart rate, pulse intensity, CRT, mucous membrane color and, often, rectal temperature. Dehydration is assessed by mucous membrane moisture, skin turgor and depth of the eyes in the socket. Perfusion deficits are in the intravascular fluid compartment. Dehydration is due to a deficit in the interstitial fluid compartment.
ii. Poor perfusion and abdominal pain. The poor perfusion is likely due to septic shock and fluid loss into the uterus and abdomen. The abdominal pain is suggestive of a peritonitis or uterine torsion.
iii. The leukopenia is of concern in the face of a probable pyometra. The dog is dehydrated, as reflected by the PCV and TS. The mild azotemia may be pre-renal, but this cannot be determined until the animal is rehydrated and the values repeated. The specific gravity was only 1.020. At this time the glucose is normal, but this must be closely monitored since septic shock increases metabolic rate. The hypokalemia will require replacement. The ACT is short, and with the mild decrease in platelets, we are concerned about early hypercoagulability. The ATIII is low, implying either loss (2+ protein in the urine) or consumption.
iv. The dog is placed on flow-by oxygen until nasal oxygen is placed. It receives 1 liter of lactated Ringer's and 500 ml of hetastarch rapidly. Butorphanol is administered as an analgesic. Then the dog is maintained on 300 ml/hr of lactated Ringer's and 300 ml/hr of hetastarch. Intravenous cefazolin, metronidazole and gentamicin are given once the dog is rehydrated. Potassium is added to the maintenance lactated Ringer's once the initial bolus is given and the blood pressure is elevated.
v. The dog should have surgery as soon as the blood pressure is between 80 and 100 mmHg MAP and central venous pressure is above 5 cmH_2O. The focus of the infection must be removed as quickly as possible to decrease the systemic exposure to cytokines. Often animals in septic shock cannot be stabilized until the focus is removed.
vi. Extreme care is taken during removal of the uterus to avoid rupturing it or allowing further leakage of purulent material. Copious lavage with body temperature sterile saline is required after removal. This dog was lavaged with 4 liters of sterile saline. The abdomen should be left open for drainage and a feeding tube placed. Cultures should be taken of the peritoneal surface prior to lacing the abdomen and sterile bandaging for the open abdomen.
vii. Fluid balance, oncotic pull, albumin, blood pressure, cardiac rate and contractility, renal function, red blood cells, oxygenation and ventilation, electrolytes and acid–base, GI function, nutrition, liver function, immune status and antibiotic selection, drug dosage and metabolism, bandages and wound care, nursing care, coagulation, mentation and glucose levels, pain management, and tender loving care.

222 First - b and e; second - d; third - a; fourth - c.

Abbreviations

ACT	Activated clotting time	ICP	Intracranial pressure
ACTH	Adrenocorticotropin hormone	IMHA	Immune-mediated hemolytic anemia
ALT	Alanine aminotransferase		
ARDS	Acute respiratory distress syndrome	IVP	Intravenous pyelogram
		LRS	Lactated Ringer's solution
ASPT	One-stage prothrombin time	MAP	Mean arterial pressure
ATIII	Antithrombin III	MCV	Mean corpuscular volume
AV	Atrioventricular	NSAID	Non-steroidal anti-inflammatory drug
BP	Blood pressure		
BUN	Blood urea nitrogen	OE	Orthopedic examination
CBC	Complete blood count	PCV	Packed cell volume
CNS	Central nervous system	PCWP	Pulmonary capillary wedge pressure
CPCR	Cardiopulmonary cerebral resuscitation		
		PT	Prothrombin time
CPP	Cerebral perfusion pressure	PTT	Partial thromboplastin time
CPR	Cardiopulmonary resuscitation	PTE	Pulmonary thromboembolism
CRI	Constant rate infusion	RBC	Red blood cells
CRT	Capillary refill time	RER	Resting energy requirement
CSF	Cerebrospinal fluid	RR	Respiratory rate
CVP	Central venous pressure	SAP	Serum alkaline phosphatase
DBP	Diastolic blood pressure	SARD	Sudden acquired retinal degeneration
DCM	Dilated cardiomyopathy		
DIC	Disseminated intravascular coagulation	SG	Specific gravity
		SIRS	Systemic inflammatory response syndrome
DPL	Diagnostic peritoneal lavage		
ECG	Electrocardiogram	SVR	Systemic vascular resistance
EG	Ethylene glycol	SVT	Supraventricular tachycardia
FDPs	Fibrin degradation products	TPR	Temperature/pulse/respiration
FeLV	Feline leukemia virus	TS	Total solids
FIP	Feline infectious peritonitis	TSH	Thyroid-stimulating hormone
FIV	Feline immunodeficiency virus	VPC	Ventricular premature contraction
GGT	Gamma glutamyl transferase	VWD	Von Willebrand's disease
GI	Gastrointestinal tract	VWF	Von Willebrand's factor
HCM	Hypertrophic cardiomyopathy	WBC	White blood cells
HR	Heart rate		

Index

All references are to question and answer numbers.

A
Abdominal counterpressure, 63, 66, 111, 123, 124
Abdominal distension, 74, 77, 106, 146, 169
Abdominal pain, 46, 87, 91, 221
Acetabular fracture, 20
Acetaminophen intoxication, 2
Acidosis
  metabolic, 54, 189
  respiratory, 149
Acute abdomen, 102
Acute tubular necrosis, 122
Addison's disease (hypoadrenocorticism), 34, 60
Advanced life support, 111
Airway obstruction, upper, 71
Albumin, 51, 186
Amputation, traumatic, 45
Analgesia, 64, 96
  pre-emptive, 64, 86
Anaphylaxis, 135
Anemia, 69, 119, 194, 210, 214
  immune-mediated hemolytic (IMHA), 7, 12, 27, 69, 206
Angioedema, 135
Antibiotics, 17, 35, 49, 126, 129
Anticholinergic drugs, 23
Antiemetics, 23, 83
Antithrombin III (ATIII), 85, 164, 192
Anuria, 87, 183
Aorta
  cross-clamping, 68
  ligation, 139
  thromboembolism, 165
Aortic insufficiency, 29
Apomorphine, 58
Arginine, 26, 52
Arrhythmias, 42, 57, 65, 146, 169
Arterial bleeding, 45, 107
Asthma, feline, 171, 211
Atlantoaxial instability/luxation, 19
Atrial fibrillation, 146
Atrioventricular (AV) block, 142, 180
Atropine, 111
Autoagglutination, 27
Autotransfusion, 70
Azotemia, 61, 122, 174, 203

B
Basic life support, 111

Bite wounds, 115, 141, 192
Blepharospasm, 53, 107, 143
Blindness, 33, 81, 104, 160
Blood, whole, 205, 209, 210
Blood pressure monitoring, 128
Blood transfusion, 70, 119, 210, 214
  reactions, 18
Bone tumors, 207
Bowel
  obstruction, 44, 212
  perforated, 197
Burns
  electrical, 170
  thermal, 15, 84, 127, 152

C
Calcitonin, 134, 182
Calcium therapy, 16, 60, 189
Caloric requirements, 43, 50
Caloric test, 219
Carbon dioxide tension (PCO_2), 124, 149
Carbon monoxide poisoning, 84, 216
Cardiac tamponade, 79, 92
Cardiomyopathy, 165
  boxer, 65
  dilated, 106, 146, 180, 195
  hypertrophic, 131
Cardiopulmonary cerebral resuscitation (CPCR), 111
Cardiopulmonary resuscitation (CPR), 6, 47, 111
  open chest, 68, 102, 111
Carnitine, 26
Carpal joints, ligamentous injuries, 94
Cellulitis, 31, 82
Central venous pressure (CVP), 75, 144
Cervical spine trauma, 19
Cesarian section, 100
Charcoal, activated, 58, 148
Chest trauma, 22, 31, 36, 156, 199
Chlorpromazine, 23
Chocolate toxicity, 148
Chorioretinitis, 160
Chylothorax, 55
Coma, 219
Compartment syndrome, 9
Consciousness, 219
Corneal injuries, 143
Corticosteroids, 21, 34, 150, 167, 211
Coughing, 76, 103, 124, 146, 171, 198, 220
Creatinine, urine:plasma ratio, 87

Cruciate ligament rupture, 14
Cushing's disease, 67
Cyanosis, 8, 73, 103

D
DAMNIT mnemonic, 41
Debridement, wound, 115, 120
Decerebrate rigidity, 219
Dehydration, 28, 60, 88, 98, 164, 173, 221
Dens, absence of, 19
Desmopressin (DDAVP), 10
Dextran-40, 4, 51, 186, 205
Dextran-70, 51, 186, 201, 205
Dextrose solutions, 87, 90, 201
Diabetes insipidus, 166
Diabetic ketoacidosis, 40, 110, 194
Diaphragmatic hernia, 140
Diaphragmatic tears, 95, 176
Diarrhea, 24, 54, 90, 91, 105, 173, 185
Diazepam, 26, 89
Diazoxide, 151
Diets, 26, 43, 50
Digoxin, 180
Disseminated intravascular coagulation (DIC), 77, 85, 162, 192
Dobutamine, 146, 157, 195
Dopamine, 111, 122, 157
Doppler blood pressure monitor, 128
Drains, wound, 132, 141
Dyspnea, 42, 55, 76, 146, 154, 206, 211, 220
Dystocia, 100

E
Eclampsia, 16
Ehrlichiosis, canine, 38
Electrical shock, 170
Emetics, 58
Endocarditis, bacterial, 29, 34
Endometritis, 122, 168
Energy requirements, 43, 50
Enteral feeding, 43, 44, 50, 52, 98, 109, 125, 132, 178
Epinephrine, 38, 111, 171
Epistaxis, 18, 38, 59
Esophageal foreign body, 178
Esophagostomy tube, 50, 109
Estrogen excess, 179, 214
Ethylene glycol (EG) toxicosis, 181
Eye trauma, 11, 143

F
Fasciitis, 31, 82
Feline leukemia virus(FeLV), 119

Feline panleukopenia, 88
Flail chest, 36
Foreign bodies, 22, 44, 53, 178, 212, 217
Fractures, 20
  failed fixation, 213
  open, 56, 113, 115, 190
Frostbite, 159
Furosemide, 39, 122, 124, 131, 134, 182, 191, 195

G
Gastric dilatation/volvulus, 74, 117, 137, 169, 200
Gastric lavage, 58
Gastric outflow obstruction, 147
Gastric ulceration, 150
Gastritis, uremic, 83
Gastroenteritis, hemorrhagic, 54
Gastropexy procedures, 117
Gastrostomy tube, 43, 50
Gelatins, 51, 186, 205
Gentamicin, 122
Glaucoma, 5, 33
Glutamine, 52
Gunshot wounds, 9, 56, 123

H
Haemobartonella felis, 119
Head injuries, 4, 62, 80, 124, 219
Heart failure, 39, 146, 154, 195, 220
Heartworm caval syndrome, 121
Heat stroke, 164
Hemangiosarcoma, 77, 193
Hematoma, 9, 13, 48
Hematuria, 48
Hemoglobinuria, 121
Hemolysis, zinc-induced, 112
Hemolytic anemia, immune-mediated (IMHA), 7, 12, 27, 69, 206
Hemophilia, 18
Hemorrhage, 10, 45, 72, 108, 139
  intra-abdominal, *see* Intra-abdominal hemorrhage
  spontaneous, 59, 118, 133
Hemothorax, 22, 70, 101, 199
Heparin, 7, 85, 165
Hepatic encephalopathy, 41
Hepatic lipidosis, 26, 50
Hepatorenal syndrome, 87
Hetastarch, 4, 51, 88, 90, 186, 201, 205
Hydrogen peroxide, 58

Hyperadrenocorticism, 67
Hypercalcemia, 1, 134, 182
Hyperglycemia, 40, 110, 203
Hyperkalemia, 34, 60, 183
Hypernatremia, 87, 153, 166
Hypersensitivity, 18, 135
Hypertension, 67, 104, 124
Hyperthermia, 164, 184
Hyperthyroidism, 42
Hypoadrenocorticism, 34, 60
Hypoaldosteronism, 60
Hypocalcemia, 16, 189
Hypokalemia, 26, 40, 110, 185
Hyponatremia, 110
Hypophosphatemia, 26, 40, 43, 194
Hypotension, 124, 157, 172
Hypotensive resuscitation, 128, 204
Hypothermia, 159
Hypoxemia/hypoxia, 118, 124, 149, 190

I
Insect stings/bites, 71, 135
Insulinoma, 151
Insulin therapy, 40, 60, 110, 183
Intercostal nerve block, 3, 30
Intervertebral disc disease, 25, 167
Intoxications, 2, 58, 112, 134, 148, 181
Intra-abdominal hemorrhage, 85, 174, 193, 196, 197
  traumatic, 63, 66, 70, 101, 114, 123, 204, 210
Intracardiac route, 111
Intracranial pressure (ICP), 124
Intraocular pressure, raised, 5, 33
Intraosseous (i/o) route, 88, 111
Intratracheal route, 111
Intussusception, 105
Ipecac, syrup of, 58

J
Jejunostomy, 109

K
Ketoacidosis, diabetic, 40, 110, 194

L
Labour, obstructed, 100
Lactated Ringer's solution (LRS), 40, 88, 90, 110, 201
Lactic acidosis, 54
Lameness, 14, 94, 138, 187, 207, 208

Laparotomy, exploratory, 43, 114, 196, 212
Large bowel disease, 24
Laryngeal paralysis, 73, 145
Lens, anterior luxation, 33
Lidocaine, 64, 106, 111, 169
Ligamentous injuries, 14, 94
Liver
  disease, 26, 41, 50, 67, 87, 185
  hemorrhage, 114, 204
  trauma, 95, 204
Local anesthetic block, 3, 30
Lung
  injuries, 199
  torsion of middle lobe, 3
Lymphoma, malignant, 182
Lymphosarcoma, 76

M
Mannitol, 4, 122, 124
Mastitis, 129
Mediastinal mass, 76
Methemoglobinemia, 2
Minithoracotomy, 68
Mitral regurgitation, 29, 154, 220
Mouth-to-nose ventilation, 188, 202
Mucous membrane color, 163
Murmurs, heart, 29, 39, 121, 154, 195

N
Nasogastric tube feeding, 50
Near-drowning, 202
Nitroglycerine, 131, 195
Nitroprusside, 195
Non-steroidal anti-inflammatory drugs (NSAIDs), 138, 150, 205
Nosocomial infections, 17
Nutritional support, 26, 43, 44, 50, 52, 98
  see also Enteral feeding
Nystagmus, 218, 219

O
Oliguria, 122, 172, 183
Osteomyelitis, fungal, 207
Osteosarcoma, 207
Oxygen
  supplementation, 101, 144, 216
  tension, arterial (PaO_2), 124, 149

P
Pain sensation, deep, 167
Pancreatitis, 51, 132, 157, 158

191

Pancytopenia, tropical, 38
Panosteitis, 138
Parenteral nutrition, 125, 132
Paresis/paralysis, 165, 167
Patellar reflex, 25, 175
Penetrating injuries, 22, 217
Penrose drains, 141
Pentastarch, 186
Pentobarbital, 89
Perfusion parameters, 221
Pericardial effusion, 79, 92
Pericardiocentesis, 92
Perineal reflex, 175
Peritoneal dialysis, 189
Peritoneal lavage, diagnostic (DPL), 174, 197
Peritonitis, septic, 85, 91, 136, 197
Petechiae, 133, 179
Phenobarbital, 89
Platelet abnormalities, 133
Pleural effusion, 126
Pneumonia, aspiration, 49
Pneumoperitoneum, 203
Pneumothorax, 22, 30, 101, 156
   tension, 68, 144
Polydipsia/polyuria, 1, 34, 40, 42, 110, 166, 182
Post-partum period, 168
Potassium therapy, 40, 194
Primary survey, 144, 163
Pringle maneuver, 114
Proptosis, traumatic, 11
Prostatitis, acute bacterial, 35
Pulmonary thromboembolism (PTE), 7, 158, 206
Pulsus paradoxus, 79
Pupillary responses, 219
Pyelonephritis, acute, 46
Pyometra, 61, 221
Pyothorax, 126
Pyuria, 46

R
Rattlesnake bites, 130
Renal failure, 183
   acute, 122, 172, 173
Renal failure
   chronic, 83, 104, 177
Renal transplantation, 177
Renal trauma, 48
Respiratory distress, 8, 47, 97, 154, 171
Respiratory distress syndrome, acute (ARDS), 82
Retinal degeneration, sudden acquired (SARD), 81

Retinal detachment, 104, 160
Rodenticide ingestion, 59, 118, 134, 198
Roundworms, 88

S
Saline (NaCl)
   0.9% (normal), 60, 147, 201
   hypertonic, 4, 90, 116
Schiff–Sherrington syndrome, 21
Sciatic nerve reflex, 175
Secondary survey, 144, 163
Sedation, 96
Seizures, 37, 41, 89, 124, 184, 222
Sepsis, 52, 141, 172, 192, 221
Sertoli cell tumors, 179
Shearing injuries, 99
Shock, 22, 96, 114, 132, 157, 191
   compensatory, 51, 66, 71, 163, 204, 221
   decompensatory, 163, 169, 185, 190
   early decompensatory (middle stage), 4, 62, 113, 115, 163
Small bowel
   anastomosis, 44
   disease, 24
Smoke inhalation, 84, 216
Snake bites, 71, 130
Sodium bicarbonate, 40, 60, 111, 189
Sodium phosphate, 194
Spherocytosis, 69
Spinal injuries, 21, 175, 215
Spleen
   enlarged, 77, 78
   ruptured, 95, 193, 209
   torsion, 78
Starvation, 98
Status epilepticus, 89
Stridor, 73, 97, 145
Stupor, 93, 181, 219
Sublingual route, 111
Systemic inflammatory response syndrome (SIRS), 12, 31, 52, 82, 101, 157, 164

T
Taurine, 26
Testicular tumors, 179, 214
Thermal injuries, 15, 84, 127, 152, 216
Thiamine, 26, 50
Third body space fluid loss, 51, 88, 90, 91

Thoracocentesis, 3, 55, 62, 126, 156, 199
Thoracostomy tube, 30, 149
Thoracotomy, 3, 68
Thrombocytopenia, 133
Thrombolytic therapy, 165
Thyroid storm, 42
Tibial crest avulsion, 208
Tourniquets, 45, 108
Trachea, collapsing, 103
Tracheotomy, 97
Transport, 6, 108, 130, 188
Triage, 32, 113, 163, 222
Tropical pancytopenia, 38

U
Unconsciousness, 188, 219
Urethral obstruction, 13, 32, 161
Urinary tract obstruction, 13, 32, 116, 161
Urine output, 183
Uroperitoneum, 197
Uterine prolapse, 155
Uveitis, acute, 107

V
Vaginal discharge, 61, 100, 162, 168, 221
Vascular occlusion/ligation, 72, 139
Ventilation, mechanical, 149
Ventricular fibrillation, 102
Ventricular premature contractions (VPCs), 169
Ventricular tachycardia, paroxysmal, 106
Vestibular disorders, 218
Viper snake bite, 71
Vitamin E, 26
Vitamin K1, 26, 59, 198
Vomiting, 28, 44, 50, 78, 83, 87, 113, 212
   center, medullary, 23
   and diarrhea, 90, 91, 105, 157, 173, 185, 201
   induction, 58
Vomitus, appearance of, 23
Von Willebrand's disease (VWD), 10, 162

W
Warfarin, 7, 59, 165
Water deficit, 166
Weight loss, 26, 29, 38, 40, 50

Z
Zinc, 26, 112